KEITH CASTLE
My second chance

To I and JP.

KEITH CASTLE

My second chance

Foreword by Eric Morecambe

PSL Patrick Stephens, Cambridge

© Keith Castle 1983

First published in 1983

British Library Cataloguing in Publication Data

Castle, Keith
My second chance.
1. Heart—Transplantation—Patients—Biography
I. Title
617'.4120592'0924   RD598

ISBN 0-85059-661-0

*Whilst every effort has been made to trace the copyright
holders for the photographs used in this book, in some
cases this has proved impossible.*

Photoset in 11 on 12 pt Plantin by Manuset Limited,
Baldock, Herts. Printed in Great Britain on Antique Wove
Vo 18 80 gsm, and bound, by The Garden City Press,
Letchworth, Herts, for the publishers,
Patrick Stephens Limited, Bar Hill, Cambridge,
CB3 8EL, England.

Contents

Foreword by Eric Morecambe

When Keith Castle asked me if I would write a Foreword for this splendid book, I said 'Yes' for two reasons—one, I like Keith, and two, part of the proceeds from the sale of *My Second Chance* will be going to the gamma camera fund at Papworth.

Without the miracles which are being performed at both Papworth and Harefield, Keith and I would never have met. However, the most up-to-date and expensive equipment is needed to help make these miracles possible, and this book is Keith's way of playing his part in raising funds for this vital gamma camera.

My Second Chance is both sad and humorous. It is also cheap when you consider that if you have any type of heart problem (and it could happen—you are no exception) you would like to think, as you are taken into hospital, that every amenity is ready and waiting for you. Well, in buying this book you may be helping yourself as well as others.

I would like to thank Keith for all the nice things he has said about me—they're all true!

Eric Morecambe

Preface

I had no intention at all of writing a book. Only certain circumstances have got me doing it now. Consequently, I have never kept any notes, with the result that I could be up to a year out on events that I have described and even more hopelessly out on facts and figures, but what does that matter? It may make a difference when I'm dead but while I'm alive and thoroughly enjoying life, I'm not bothered if I am a year or so out on statistics.

Professional writers may cringe at my literary style. I should worry! To me this book is written in everyday language. I've spent too much time in my life nearly 'splitting me differences' to worry about a few split infinitives.

I would have liked to have called this book *Lie back and think of English*, but I know I wouldn't have got away with it. For a start, Mr Terence English, being the type of man he is, would have had my guts for garters! If I had used this title it would have been to try to give, in a clumsy way, a message to all sick and worried patients. I was so lucky in having so much faith in everyone who helped to cure me that, honestly, all my family and I faced the operation with complete equanimity, with no worries at all. We had faith in the fact that nothing was going to go wrong. We hope that having absolutely no hang-ups was our contribution to the proceedings and helped to make it a success. If any patient can do the same thing, and view his doctor in the same light I viewed mine, he will become fully relaxed and have no worries. I think this is the part the patient must play. Therefore, he will have full confidence in his surgeon and will be able to safely 'Lie back and think of English' as I did.

1

The start of it all

If I had had the 'standard' type of heart attack, I would have turned purple in the face, have had pains across my chest, collapsed on the floor in agony and had people milling round me, alternatively giving me the kiss of life or thumping my chest! Fortunately, not all heart attacks are like that, which I suppose is my cue to tell you about my first—and very unconventional—heart attack.

'Candy, we're working too hard, so let's stop and have a cup of tea,' I said. Candy, who originally got the nickname because he happened to work on the candy floss machine in the Festival Gardens during the Festival of Britain, readily agreed. I carried on doing the plastering whilst he was making the tea.

It was Sunday morning—November 7 1976. As I was a builder by profession, I was helping Candy to build an extension at the back of his premises and, on this day, we were doing all the plastering. Being a bit of a dab hand (or so I thought) I had spread on rather a lot of plaster and this created a great deal of arm movement to get the required finish over such a large area, and, I thought, that was why I was getting so hot.

I decided to go to the front door and have a couple of breaths of fresh air. After a few minutes I realised that, having at first leant against the door, I was now sitting on the pavement. It was pouring with rain so I reasoned that one of two things was happening. Either I was ill or I was a raving lunatic. I had no chest pains at all or anything like that. It was just that I felt so extremely hot. I called to Candy to take me home.

At home I immediately went up to the bathroom to take a bath— simply because I was smothered in plaster—while Candy explained the position to Doreen, my wife, and advised her to call an ambulance. The evening before we had eaten some fish and, mindful of the fact that we are always told to be sensible, I wound Doreen up by telling her to put some sample fish in a jar to take to the hospital, just in case it was food poisoning! Doreen was more interested in getting *me* to the hospital, rather than a jar of fish, and couldn't see quite what I was talking about, but I was adamant. She did it. Anyway, the ambulance duly arrived and took us to St James's Hospital—a place with which I was to become very familiar in the ensuing years.

At St James's a quick diagnosis was made. Yes, it was a heart attack. Following the usual routine of hospitals in such cases, I was taken to the Intensive Care Unit straight away. Not feeling particularly ill, I was able to sit up and take stock of my surroundings. To my surprise, St James's Intensive Care Unit, rather than being grim and forbidding, was, on the contrary, very, very bright and cheerful looking. The next couple of hours were spent with some doctors carrying out routine tests on me and eventually I was well and truly settled in and entered on Professor Pilkington's list as his patient. Doreen visited me that evening, bringing all my requisites—toothpaste, toothbrush and pyjamas, etc—and neither of us was unduly worried because, as I have already said, I didn't feel all that bad.

I spent the next couple of days in the Intensive Care Unit and then I was transferred to Ward 1. If I said earlier that I was to become very familiar with St James's Hospital over the following years, it was Ward 1 in particular which was to become my home for the next two and a half years. (Ward 1 is a Men's Medical Ward with 36 beds.)

As you approach Ward 1, there are two single cubicles and a three-bedded cubicle before you enter the main ward. Immediately on the right is the Sister's cubicle. Three-quarters of the way down the ward there is a partition and, past this, there are a further five beds which lead off into the Day Room. The beds down the left-hand side of the ward are fitted up with oxygen apparatus—logically for people with breathing problems. A third of the way down, in the gangway, is the desk at which the night staff can sit. This has an overhead light which can be pulled down to shine directly on the top. Quite naturally, any patient who has to be watched a little more closely than the others is put near to the night staff station. My position, because of my difficulty in breathing, was the bed nearest the night staff on the oxygen side.

At that time of the year, the whole of the left-hand side of the ward was occupied with patients suffering from bronchitis, two of whom I was to get to know very well. Dick Martin had plain bronchitis. Bill Lodder had suffered severe gassing during the First World War and this had affected his chest. These two were firm friends. Over the months, two, if not three, of us found ourselves back in the ward at any one time. Dick and Bill were two of the greatest comedians I have ever met in a hospital! Even when it came to looks, if Dick Martin was Bud Flanagan, then Bill Lodder was certainly his Ches.

As a Men's Medical Ward, Ward 1 has a variety of cases. As I said previously, at that time of the year there were many bronchitic patients, but the range of illnesses also included strokes, heart attacks, diabetes, and there was always one amnesic patient and a fair smattering of junkies, attempted suicides and folk like that. Quite naturally, being new to this heart attack business, I was more interested in talking to the other heart patients in the ward. To my intense surprise and horror, some of them told me they were back in the ward following their second and third heart attacks, which I just couldn't believe. I just couldn't see that anybody could come back *again* for something like a heart attack. Surely, after the first warning shot across the bows, you would do everything in life to prevent getting another one. I was determined that this was going to be my one and only visit to hospital for a heart attack, which just goes to show what a rotten prophet I turned out to be! The rest of the week passed pleasantly enough—the food was plentiful and the company was good. I also got my first dose of Martin and Lodder's humour!

Barbara, the Ward Sister, placed an Asian gentleman between the two practical jokers, Dick Martin and Bill Lodder. (For the sake of anonymity, we had better call him Mr R.) He was one of those very, very demanding patients. He insisted on full attention for the least little thing and, if he had been allowed to, he would have taken up at least 90 per cent of the nurses' complete day. He was more interested in worrying about his grocery business than lying back in bed, doing as he was told, and trying to get better. Dozens of times a day he was on the telephone worrying about bags of Patna rice instead of his health.

On this particular day, a blood sample had been taken from him and he had been left with his finger holding a little cotton wool pad over his arm. This is the normal routine. But, in his jumping about, up and down to the telephone, he had opened up the vein and blood was spurting up in the air, like a miniature fountain. He was yelling, as usual, for attention, and the nurses, who had not spotted the blood and were by now used to him crying wolf, ignored him, and carried on attending to the other patients. As soon as Dick Martin twigged this, he was in like a bullet! He gave Bill the eye, and together they started to give Mr R. the benefit of their medical knowledge.

'Now look, mate, that little cotton wool pad will never stop your arm bleeding. There's a very special paste that they have in hospitals for that sort of thing. It's very expensive and generally they don't like letting it out—you'll have to *insist* upon it. They call it Polyfilla—but they won't give it to you unless you demand it!'

Immediately Mr R. was screaming out for Polyfilla! Naturally, the nurses, not seeing his bleeding arm and just hearing him calling out for Polyfilla, again ignored him. His demands not being met, Mr R. was gradually getting more and more agitated and excitable and, in the end, it took all Barbara's diplomacy to simmer him down. When semi-calm had been restored, Barbara rounded on the other two and gave them a wigging—but what could she do when Martin just looked sheepish and said: 'Well, it *could* have worked, couldn't it?'

I got to know Mr R. and grew to like him a lot in the next few days.

His was rather a tragic story at the finish because, on the day of his discharge from hospital, I said to his wife: 'Now look, don't let him go rushing straight into the business and worrying about the till and the takings and the rice and the flour—make him calm down.' But, early the next morning, we got the buzz that they had admitted him again to the Intensive Care Unit, where he had had another heart attack and died. He had overdone it and had returned to the rat race far too quickly.

Approaching the end of my first week in hospital, they decided to move me into the three-bedded cubicle. When Doreen and Kevin (my youngest son) came to see me on the early visit that Sunday, I just happened to mention that I really fancied one of those malt liquors—something I don't normally drink. Naturally, Kevin made it his avowed intention and ambition to treat me. On the evening visit, in he walked with six cans of malt liquor for me. After he and Doreen had gone, it didn't take us long to divide the booze up—three of us in the ward, six cans of liquor, two apiece—so we sat down and, chatting comfortably, drank them. Just after we had finished, I was sitting on my bed and the nurse came in to do the observations. To my great surprise, I got a complete loss of colour vision. Naturally, knowing the nurse, I could recognise her silhouette, but all I could see was a black figure, walking through a black door—everything black. Of course I got a bit concerned about it and I mentioned it to the nurse. She said: 'Oh, don't worry, you've probably just had a little fainting fit, lie back on your bed for a few minutes.'

After she had completed the observations and had gone, I turned to the other two and said: 'Well, I think for the rest of the night I'm getting into bed fully.' I got out of bed to take my dressing gown off and place it on what was rather a low chair . . . that is all I can remember. My next recollection was that I was lying on the floor, with a couple of nurses trying to pick me up. I didn't feel too good because, apart from fainting, in falling rather heavily I had apparently cracked my head on a locker as I had gone down. The nurses put me into bed and sent for the doctor. Just as he came through the door, I had a repeat performance of the loss of colour vision. I could recognise the doctor but, as before, I saw a black silhouette, coming through a black door. This time, however, there was a slight difference and the doctor (Dr Bellamy) marked down on the notes that I had reported a slight green haze around the silhouette. (Your first impressions are always the most accurate; later on the imagination can take over.) Dr Bellamy then gave me a quick checkover and straight away advised my transfer to the Intensive Care Unit.

Now, it's a very unfortunate fact about hospital life that, in order to avoid accusations of theft, whenever a patient goes to a different ward, or is transferred somewhere else, his gear has to go with him. It can take

1 minute to shift you up to another ward to attempt to save your life, but *2 minutes* to pack your things. It's too bad if your life depends on it—your gear must be packed *before* you can go! So, there I was, lying on a stretcher, waiting to go up to the Intensive Care Unit, and the nurses were rushing around, packing my stuff into a plastic bag.

Apparently, when I collapsed, a young boy in the ward with us flew out, in a bit of a panic, to call a nurse. On his return he saw the six empty cans of malt liquor lying about and bunged them all into my locker. Consequently, when the nurses had to pack my gear, out tumbled the six empty cans! The young lad quickly explained the true story to the doctor and, Dr Bellamy, being a good sort, turned to my worrying mate and said: 'Oh well, it's only a load of gnats' pee anyway, isn't it?'

So, it was back up to the Unit again for the second time that week. But, this time, there was a subtle difference. They put me into one of the glass cubicles, instead of the main part of the Unit. They quickly wired me up to all the monitoring machines and sent for the registrar on duty. Now the joke was, I still wasn't in any pain and, once again, I had an obsession about fish. We had had a lovely fish supper that night and I blamed my condition on this and told the doctor so. But he knew different. From this period up until about midnight, events were to move fast and furiously and I was only hazily aware of half of them. As far as I was concerned it was just a succession of lying back and going to sleep, then waking up, sitting upright and talking to the nurses and then lying back and going to sleep again. What I *didn't* realise was that, when I thought I was lying back and going to sleep, I was actually having a bad heart attack and, indeed, on a couple of these occasions I arrested. At one time I can remember sitting up in bed, talking to this gorgeous Chinese staff nurse. Suddenly, she took one look at me, her eyes as large as saucers, and then bounded out into the corridor, faster than Brendan Foster ever could make it, to fetch the doctor again. I can also remember being washed—in actual fact they had to wash my pyjamas as well because I was not in charge of all my bodily functions— but to this day I still swear blind (and I have a sneaky suspicion) that they were laying me out. I'd love to find out if they were or not!

During one of my lucid moments, the doctor said to me: 'Would you like us to send for your son?' (My eldest son, Keith). I didn't know why they should want to send for him at that time of night, but I agreed. So they phoned young Keith but, at the time, he didn't have any transport, so he ran the mile between his house and ours. He was going to tell Doreen and bring her up to the hospital somehow. However, the curtains were drawn and, not seeing any lights on, he decided that she was in bed asleep and that he would go to the hospital alone. What he *didn't* know was that some sixth sense had made Doreen get up out of bed. At that moment she was sitting downstairs by the fire. Young Kevin had woken up too, and, realising his mother was downstairs, had gone down to sit on her lap. Why Doreen did this, we don't know to this day. Neither of us are people who bother about analysing human behaviour or emotions; we let others lay claims to ESP and all that sort of thing. Indeed, if I wanted to make a claim I could have said that I saw ectoplasm, or something similar, as I looked down at my body when I was arresting—but no—there was nothing like that. The plain truth is: I was either asleep (in fact arresting) or was wide awake. It's as simple as that.

Anyway, Keith arrived at the hospital and the doctors soon put him in the picture. He stayed a few hours then went home. The next morning, having only managed to snatch a couple of hours' sleep, he went round to Doreen to tell her all about it. She went straight to the hospital. She looked for a doctor to speak to, but unfortunately didn't recognise any of them as I had only been in hospital a week. (She had, in fact, passed one of them going up the stairs, without knowing who he was.) She found a doctor and he asked her to sit down and have a cup of tea. He spoke gently to her, but eventually said: 'Look, Mrs Castle, we must start talking about possible death.' Well, of course this was a shock to Doreen, and she turned to him angrily saying: 'Don't you start talking about death as far as *he* is concerned. You've got a fighter on your hands there, and I don't think you realise it.' I am glad that she was so prophetic!

After a few more days in Intensive Care, I was transferred back to Ward 1 again where, after a couple of weeks had gone by, somebody started talking about discharge from hospital. It was to be conditional on my passing a very simple little practical test. With a couple of student doctors, I was to walk out of the ward, up a couple of flights of stairs, see if I was all right, walk back down the stairs and get back into bed. All this was duly carried out without any trouble whatsoever. But, as I was talking to the two students by my bed, while taking off my dressing gown, I suddenly experienced pains right across my shoulders. (Typical angina pains, although angina was a thing that I didn't suffer from subsequently.) I told the students that I had got these pains and, as I was talking to them, everything seemed to go wrong and I really felt terrible. They put me on the bed and then all panic broke loose. The alarm button was pressed, everybody started running, curtains were pulled around my bed, and I can remember Barbara standing at the head of the bed, holding a basin into which I was vomiting all the time. The pain was a bit strong, and it was one of the few occasions when I did have pain. The next minute I was put on to a stretcher and, as I was being wheeled out of the ward, old Lodder stood up, shook my hand and said: 'Look after yourself, boy, you've done well so far, don't

14

let it all go now.' Once again, I was back to the familiar faces and surroundings of the Intensive Care Unit.

Well, of course, on her next visit to the hospital, Doreen made a mistake which she was to repeat quite frequently in the days to come! She went into Ward 1 and, when she couldn't find me, she asked the Sister where I was. Sister told her that I was up in the Unit again, so up she came. The next time she visited me she made straight for the Intensive Care Unit—of course, this time, I was back downstairs. Again and again, she would arrive at one place, only to find out that I was at the other. The amount of time she had to spend traipsing round that place!

Anyhow, this was the period when we were approaching Christmas and, although I was in the Unit and not feeling too good, it was a nice sort of time because Doreen was planning with Sister Screech to put up little decorations, not, of course, inside the Unit, but in the corridor just outside. She was also busy deciding what decorations she was going to make for Ward 1. I could only take part in the discussions about Christmas decorations when I was 'waking up' as this was a time when I was undergoing a complete change of drugs as things weren't improving and I seemed to be going downhill only. It had been decided to try different types and amounts of drugs. This routine became very familiar to me. There would be a heavy increase in the build-up of drugs, a complete change in my body, then another heavy build-up of drugs, followed by another body change and this routine went on for months and months.

Anyway, I was eventually sent back to Ward 1 for good. That was it. I was a terminal patient. I found this out in the easiest and simplest manner going. I overheard one doctor telling another that he thought I had about two months to live. I kept stumm about it though to Doreen. Christmas was approaching fast and my only worry was whether they would allow me home for the holiday. However, Professor Pilkington immediately put the block on that. He said I might get too excited and it would be better if I waited until after the holiday.

Talking of Christmas is an ideal cue to introduce Albert—the ward's favourite patient. Albert was a very young-looking man in his middle 70s. All he had done was fall over and hit his head and was now suffering from loss of memory. The trouble with people like Albert is that there is nowhere really suitable for them to go. You can't put them into a home because they would go downhill rapidly there. Generally speaking, the hospital hangs on to people like that in the hope that something might crop up at a later stage. Poor old Albert was well and truly disorientated—the minute he moved away from his bed he was hopelessly and completely lost! He had no sense of direction whatsoever. On many occasions, Doreen would find him wandering about up the corridors, she'd see him back to his bed, turn round and walk out, and no sooner had she gone a little way up the corridor, than she would find poor old Albert following her again! No one ever knew where he was.

However, Albert's main trouble was that he was very badly incontinent. He always swore blind that the ceiling leaked and, to pacify him, they used to move him about to different positions in the ward, but to his horror, this wet patch of ceiling was always above his head! Now, if Albert became wet, he would make his way to the end of the ward and the dirty linen basket, find a pair of soiled pyjamas which had been placed there to be washed and put them on, forgetting to take the wet ones underneath off first. On other occasions he would get his suit and put it on (on top of the two pairs of pyjamas!). Even if the leg was twisted inside out, he always managed somehow to get the trousers on. Then there would be another 'accident' and Albert would again raid the linen basket, putting on a third pair of pyjamas over his suit and the first two pairs. Well, by the time Albert had put on about six outfits he began to hum a little bit, to put it mildly! Not only that, with his poor sense of direction, every time he saw an empty bed, he would just dive straight into it, much to the annoyance of the patient whose bed it was, and then all hell would break loose because the patient would insist that the sheets were changed. So, one little walk up the ward by Albert could result in the need for six beds to be stripped and then made again with clean sheets!

With Christmas approaching we decided we must find a way for Albert to find his own bed. The nurses found a huge piece of red ribbon and tied a marvellous bow on the end of his bed with it, saying: 'Albert, the bed with the Christmas bow on is yours. Please try not to get into other people's beds, you've got your own special Christmas Cracker bed now.' All this was to no avail. All the months I knew Albert, he was always bed-hopping and bed-wetting. But the marvellous thing was that he was always such a kind and gentle man. In his lucid moments he talked very intelligently. To my shame, I don't know where Albert is today—somewhere comfortable, I hope, because he thoroughly deserved it.

Christmas was spent with choirs visiting the ward, priests of all denominations popping in to see various patients and nurses distributing presents to all of us—we even had a couple of glasses of sherry! But the thing which tickled my sense of humour was that, at a quarter to one (after our lunch) Christmas was all over for us! Even though it was the festive season, we were still sick patients and so we were all packed off to bed.

After Christmas, arrangements were made for me to go home. The family began to redecorate the lounge and put a bed in there for me because, by then, I couldn't have managed the stairs. Before this work was completed, they visited me and, to their horror, were told by the new doctor who had joined us (Bill Brough), that I could come home

16

the following day. The family had a quick word with him in the corridor, explaining that the lounge wasn't quite ready. Dr Brough promised to stall me for the next two or three days. He came and told me he'd rather keep me in for a few more days, and I fell for it. Barbara, in the meantime, had told Professor Pilkington about the arrangements, but we hadn't taken the Professor's puckish sense of humour into account. At rounds the next day he turned to Dr Brough at my bedside and said: 'I think this patient can go home tomorrow, don't you?' Broughie, not wanting to let on in front of me about the room being re-decorated, disagreed with the Professor, which is very unusual for a houseman. Well, of course, the more he disagreed with the Prof, the more the Prof started getting at him! 'What is the basis of your diagnosis when you say he cannot go home tomorrow, when *I* say he can go home?' asked the Professor. To give Broughie his due, he stuck to his guns and I don't think to this day that he has ever lost out for having had the courage to stand his ground. I also feel certain that he never knew that the Professor knew all about his plan with my family to keep me in for a few more days.

A couple of days later, Doreen picked me up. We packed my gear and home we went. The first thing that jumped up and licked my face was the present which the family had bought me—a lovely little Jack Russell puppy called Lady. The idea was that she would keep me company. It was a very nice, quiet, little episode in my life, but it didn't last for long.

2

Early St James's

I forget what caused my next admittance to St James's Hospital, but I seemed to be continually in and out of that place for several months. At least it gave me the opportunity to renew my acquaintance with Dick Martin and Bill Lodder, to say nothing of being able to follow the continuing saga of Albert and the wet patches of ceiling which followed him from bed to bed!

It was at this time that I found out a golden rule of hospital life. (I should say it became *my* golden rule of hospital life.) Doreen had decided to buy me a pair of moccasin slippers. They were very nice but, of course, they didn't actually have leather soles. Unfortunately, in a large ward where there seemed to be a good number of incontinent old chaps, the toilet floors were usually awash with urine because many of them got 'caught short'. I soon learned that the soft-soled moccasins soaked this up like a sponge! Needless to say, I quickly discarded them and from then on I never wore moccasin type slippers in a hospital.

One group of patients in the ward were diabetics. Now they carried out a slightly different routine from everybody else. They had to have a test first thing in the morning and again last thing at night. Because, except for their diabetes, they were fit and active people, there was a general rule that they should stay in hospital for the night, following their late night test, have their morning test and then were free to do almost anything they liked during the day. Many of them used to go out to work.

One day, Dick Martin and Bill Lodder wanted to place a bet. Cathy, who usually did this for us, had the day off, so they asked a diabetic patient if he would mind going up to the local betting shop and putting the bet on for them. He replied that he would be delighted, as it would give him something to do. So, the boys made out their slip and, at lunch time, out he went. They heard on the radio that their horses had won, but there was no sign of the diabetic fellow, and they wondered if he had run off with their winnings. Anyhow, late in the evening, he arrived back in the ward very merry or, more accurately, very drunk!

'What on earth has happened to you?' asked Dick and Bill. 'Well, to be honest,' was the reply, 'although I said I would put your bets on for you, I had never been into a betting shop before in my life and, because *The County Arms* was next door to the shop, I popped in there to fortify myself with a couple of drinks.'

He had liked the atmosphere in the betting shop so much that he had spent the afternoon going from one establishment to another and, when the pub closed for the afternoon, he went straight back to the first shop. He decided to wait for the announcement of the winners of the last race and then went into the pub, which had re-opened by then, and all in all he had thoroughly enjoyed his day! I can't ever remember Cathy putting on another bet for us, as our friendly diabetic was always the first volunteer thereafter!

One day, dear old Albert excelled himself. He saw a familiar figure walking out of the ward and decided to follow, complete with his full wet regalia. Somehow, he managed to get right out of the hospital grounds, still following the bloke who was heading towards the infamous betting shop. Unfortunately, half way up the road, Albert lost sight of him, which was probably just as well because I can imagine the confusion that Albert would have caused in a bookie's! Anyway, back at the hospital, the hue and cry was raised. They were well used to Albert wandering about the buildings or grounds, but the fact that he was nowhere to be found threw them into a panic. Eventually, poor old Albert was found walking around aimlessly—presumably looking for a spare bed to climb into!

Easter 1977 was a rotten period for me. I did nothing but vomit. It used to be so embarrassing when I was out shopping with Doreen. By then, I couldn't go more than 30 yards for several reasons—a) because of the weakness in my legs, b) because of my difficulty in breathing and c) because I had the continual embarrassment of, every few yards, having to turn round to find a nice quiet little corner to vomit in. Eventually, I gave up going out altogether. Soon enough, I was taken back into St James's to find out why I was vomiting so much.

At first, they talked about a hiatus hernia, but there was the possibility that I had a duodenal ulcer. There was only one way to find out—more tests. Well, I had a barium meal test which confirmed what they called a 'chronic duodenal'; I remember the lady who carried out the tests expressing surprise when I said I was vomiting, but not in pain. The next day, I was due to go down to confirm this diagnosis, which involved a test where they put an optic fibre down your throat to have a butchers at your tummy.

St James's were very proud of their Examination Unit. I think they considered that it was the best one in Europe. They have about six to nine beds (depending on the number of patients they have at one session) and these are arranged in a crescent formation. At the top of the crescent are two rooms. One is the preparatory room and the other room is the operating room—so that the patient in bed number one gets into the preparatory room first, then the operating room. By the time everyone had been seen, the first patient had had a couple of hours sleep to recover, and, if he was an out-patient, was able to go home.

As I was an 'in-patient', I wasn't due to go down until just before lunch time, probably to be the last of the day's session, so it was a complete surprise to everybody when, early on in the morning, a porter came into the ward to take me to the theatre. I had been caught out on the hop and decided I wanted a quick cigarette before I went down there. I said to Barbara: 'Oh, Barbara—I can't go down to theatre so quickly just like this. I must use the loo before I go.' She said I could have a quick visit to the loo, and told me to take my surgical gown and change in there! It seemed very incongruous to me as I had a quick drag on my fag and got into my sterile equipment in the loo, then hurried back into the ward and jumped on to the stretcher on the trolley.

Barbara decided to accompany me, with my notes, to the operating theatre. It was a fairly long walk from our ward. On the way down, I could see Barbara arguing with the porter, but I couldn't hear what the argument was. Eventually, things got a bit heated, and when the trolley had stopped at an intersection of corridors, I asked Barbara what on earth was going on. She told me that there was a porters' and technicians' strike later on that day, and the porter was arguing the toss as to whether or not I was an emergency patient, because I happened to be already inside the hospital. Barbara said she was busy telling him that due to the number of times I had collapsed in front of her nurses I was *definitely* an emergency patient.

Anyway, we carried on down to the Unit and I took my place in the crescent-shaped queue of beds, awaiting my turn to have the examination. Some time went by and then the consultant in charge of the Unit put his head round the door and said to the nurse: 'That Professor Pilkington patient—will he be long?' The nurse replied that I was there, but would be quite some time getting to him as I was at the back of the queue. He asked her to put me forward next because at lunch time there was to be a consultants' meeting to see what was happening with the strike and that he wanted at that time to confirm my diagnosis to Professor Pilkington. So I was next in the queue.

I went into the pre-med room, where the anaesthetist explained that he would first of all give me a small dose of the anaesthetic and then, just before I went into the operating room, he would give me a full shot of the drug. He duly gave me the preliminary dose and, whilst I was lying there, the technician came in from the other room, looked round and went back into the theatre. Then I had the full dose. No sooner had this full dose been administered, than the technician decided that he was going to join the strike. Had he made up his mind 10 seconds

20

earlier, I wouldn't have had the full dose. So there was I, going out like a light, and the examination had been aborted! I was then wheeled back to Ward 1.

I heard later, on good authority, that over the lunchtime period, when Professor Pilkington heard about what had happened to me, he went hopping mad. He gave the shop steward a good going over and told him that his strikers had put the life of his patient in jeopardy. Consequently, I had to go down to theatre again in the afternoon and go through it all again. It was a funny little type of test. I can remember they put a thing very similar to a cotton reel between my teeth, then wound a scarf around my head so that I was biting on it. Presumably, this was done to stop me biting my tongue or something. They then fed a tube down my throat through the hole in the middle of this reel. Anyway, it only confirmed what everyone had known from the previous day's examination—it was a chronic duodenal ulcer.

When the results came to the ward, Broughie was on duty, and it was his job to prescribe some medicine for the ulcer. He then rang someone to check on this. (I assume that it was the laboratory.) The next day, they delivered this medicine and I can only describe it as being 99 per cent ammonia as a solvent for the 1 per cent of whatever it was that cured the ulcer. It was also an awkward thing to take from a timing point of view, because I could only take it up to half an hour before meals, or half an hour after meals. Apparently, the way it worked was that it went down, slowly spread over the ulcer and formed a protective skin, and any foods or liquids that were taken down *while* the medicine was actually forming the skin would actually melt away. But, of course, I was also on massive amounts of pills which had to be taken at certain times before, and certain times after, meals so between it all it was like a clockwork routine which couldn't be deviated from for a minute. Apart from this, the medicine was horrible to take!

On the next full doctor's round, with everybody there, the Professor asked me what the medicine was like. 'Oh, it's all right,' I said, 'if you bear in mind it seems to be 99 per cent ammonia, so it's not very pleasant to take.' Allan Cleary, the Senior Registrar, immediately panicked, assuming that I could have had a batch of medicine which had gone off. He flew to the telephone to check with the drug manufacturers but they confirmed that that was the taste of it.

At this stage, the Professor's puckish sense of humour again came into play. He made a great fuss about the cost of the medicine (which was £10 a bottle) although he knew this was for a 28-day supply. He asked Broughie if he had checked up on the use of expensive medicines and Broughie replied that he only prescribed what the lab had suggested. The Prof then suggested that Broughie should taste every medicine that he prescribed. Having heard my description of the taste,

21

Broughie steeled himself, but did in fact take a spoonful. He nearly vomited at the taste! Of course, I kept getting at him for the rest of the day!

Now Broughie was actually a very good cricketer, but I used to gee him up that this was a load of old rubbish! I always issued the challenge to him that I would let him have six bowls at me down the length of the ward. He could use any ball he liked—I would only use a bed bottle— and I would definitely hit six consecutive sixes off him! But he never took up the challenge.

It was decided that I could go home to allow the ulcer to have its full 28-day cure. I rang Doreen to ask her to bring me some clothes, which she duly did. I pulled the curtains round my bed whilst I got changed. Shirt, underpants, vest, tie, socks—everything but trousers! She had forgotten my trousers! I can remember having to wait in the hospital, until she had gone all the way home to fetch a pair for me!

I remember that, before the 28-day treatment for the ulcer was up, I was admitted back into St James's again. But the treatment did work and it kept the ulcer at bay—let's put it that way!

One Saturday, whilst I was in there, they decided to scrub the ward floor. The place was full of visitors. Doreen, of course, was with me. The scrubbing operation was planned down to the last minute. They were going to push all the beds, patients, visitors, everything, to one side of the ward and scrub the other side, dry it out and polish it and then reverse the procedure. As you know, the best laid plans never work out! There was total confusion everywhere. I took one look at Broughie and said: 'And you say I'm supposed to have complete bed rest! What, with all this going on?' He agreed it was ridiculous and suggested that I might like to go home for the weekend. 'Yes, please,' I replied very promptly! 'Clear off then,' he said, 'and don't come back until Monday morning so we can get the ward cleaned and polished for you.'

I think it was on this visit that Doreen was in for a shock. She tripped into Sister's office to pick up my usual fortnightly sick certificate. Sister wrote one out for three months and Doreen said: 'Sister, there's some mistake here. You've given me a 13 week certificate, and usually it's only for two.' Barbara looked at Doreen in surprise. 'My dear,' she said, 'hasn't one of the doctors told you?' 'Told me what?' asked Doreen. 'I'm afraid that Keith will never be able to go to work again. All he can do now is go home and do some of his paintings.' 'My God,' said Doreen, 'I can't tell him that. I think you had better come out and tell him this.' So the two of them came out and sat on my bed. Barbara started talking to me about painting—which she knew was my great hobby—and she tried to let me down lightly. This episode confirmed what Doreen had suspected for some time, but which I had known for quite a long while—that I was slowly but surely going downhill.

22

There followed, in quick succession, two amusing little incidents which certainly broke up the monotony of hospital life. The first was that, half way down the ward, I noticed that the curtains were continuously drawn around a bed, and to me that rang a bell that the patient had died. They were obviously going to leave him until the evening, when we were all bedded down, and then they would screen off all the beds and move the body out. Well, during the course of that evening when I was in the rest room, the nurses asked us to go back to our beds and get bedded down. We knew what it was—they wanted to screen off. 'Oh hell,' we moaned, 'there's a good programme on TV—can't we stay and watch it?' 'All right then,' they said, 'provided you stay in there and shut the door.' We agreed. When our programme had finished we were all ready for bed. The morticians hadn't come in yet, so we crept back to our various beds, and the nurses pulled our curtains. Well, one little nurse had to do an observation on me. She came into my cubicle and did this but, on going out, she forgot to pull the curtains. Eventually, in came the morticians. They put the body in the coffin and were just wheeling it out when they came level with my bed and saw me sitting up with an amused look on my face, watching it all go on! It was the nurse who nearly had a heart attack when she saw me!

The next day, an old chap was admitted who wasn't ill at all. However, he was 83 and his wife was ill, and the poor old fellow was so lost without her that, while she was in the hospital in another ward being attended to, they decided to put him in Ward 1 to be looked after as there was nowhere else for him to go. He wanted to spend every minute with his wife, and the nurse had to spend a lot of the time taking him up to the other ward every time he asked. That evening, he couldn't understand why he couldn't be with his wife and had to go to bed with us in Ward 1. He was getting rather irascible about this and he picked an argument with another patient in our ward who was 81. Anyhow, tempers were flying and the next minute the two old chaps were throwing punches at each other! Well, there was a crowd of nurses at the far end of the ward and one called Sue walked down the ward to separate them. It was quite a mild affair, so none of the other nurses even bothered to give Sue a hand. Sue took the arm of the old chap of 83 and gently started guiding him back to his bed. Then he started wrestling with *her*! Well, there's an old saying that the madman has the strength of ten. Whether or not he had gone momentarily mad, I don't know, but he certainly seemed to have more strength than Sue, who was, in fact, a big strapping girl. Gradually, he bent her backwards over the bed. Having forced her right down, he began slowly to try to get on top of her. To all intents and purposes he appeared to be raping her! Of course, nothing like that was going on—in fact Sue was killing herself with laughter and the other nurses at the other end of the ward were hysterical! No one moved to help poor Sue and she had to get out of the situation as best she could! I accused her for months after that she was bitterly disappointed that things had not taken their natural course!

Eventually, calm was again restored and Sue went back to join the other giggling nurses. However, the old chap was not finished yet. He immediately turned on poor Mr Gossai, an amnesic patient who had taken old Albert's place in the ward. Like Albert, he was a kind and gentle man but, having had a stroke, he had no use in his right arm at' all. When the old chap picked on him, the kind and gentle Gossai was at first terrified. He backed off from the man, but thrust out his left arm as a jab . . . it turned out to be an excellent jab—far better than Henry Cooper ever had!

At last we separated them and Gossai, who was still frightened, took some calming down. I tried to cheer him up by saying I would become his manager and make him a world champion boxer within 12 months. Gradually, he lost his fear and saw the funny side of things. He was, by nature, a very quiet chap and his daily ritual consisted of buying his cigarettes and matches, for which he had just enough pocket money. He had a speech impediment, because of his stroke and so he would ask, by tapping his pocket which held this money, one of the other patients to buy these things, and he would then spend the whole day in the television room. His greatest achievement was to watch a marathon showing of the Pope's investiture. Being Asian, he understood little of the proceedings, but he watched hour after hour, as cardinals knelt before the Pope and kissed his hand. He didn't understand a word of it, but he kept on watching.

About this time, Dick Martin ran a sweepstake for the Derby. He touted everybody in the ward to take part—from Professor Pilkington downwards. Everyone drew a piece of paper out of a hat which gave them the name of their horse. The television room was crowded whilst the Derby was being run, and we all cheered for our own horse. Everyone was surprised when Dick Martin's horse, My Love, won. Right from the beginning there had been jokes about the fiddling going on. Dick looked the picture of innocence and said, with his hand on his heart, that it was all above board, and no one could argue with him! I had my doubts! I must say though, he wouldn't fiddle a thing like that for financial reasons—he would do it for a giggle. He was most generous and was always chipping into some ward kitty or other.

I don't remember how long I spent in hospital on that occasion, but I was eventually discharged. The same old thing happened again. I started vomiting continually. It was the bane of my life, not only embarrassing for me, but for Doreen as well, but she always put on a very brave face. At this time, I remember occasions when I would be lying in bed and I'd hear Doreen creeping up the stairs to put her head round the door to see whether or not I was still breathing. This went on until July 1977 when the next major event occurred.

I was back at St James's. It was a Saturday morning and the patients were all sitting round the breakfast table. I turned to the chaps and said: 'Gentlemen, I don't think I feel like any breakfast this morning, I'm going back to bed.' One of them looked up in alarm and said: 'What's the matter, Keith, don't you feel very well?' 'No,' I replied, 'I'm not in any pain, but I just feel a bit rough,' and I duly crept back to bed and went to sleep.

I woke up to the strangest sensation of being pulled through the air. This was actually happening because two orderlies were lifting me from the bed on to a stretcher, with Broughie standing by, leaning over me. He looked down and said to me: 'Don't worry, Mr Castle, the Intensive Care Unit is almost empty, so I thought you could have a nice quiet weekend up there.' In actual fact, Broughie suspected that I had suffered a pulmonary embolus. Up to the Unit I went, where tests showed that, yes, Broughie was correct. There was more than one occasion when Broughie saved my life with a bit of quick thinking.

Now followed a sad little incident. The day before, I said to Doreen: 'Look, love, you have been visiting me every single day for ages and ages. Have a day off tomorrow.' Doreen, who was very tired, agreed. Anyway, when she came up to see me on the Sunday, she made the usual mistake. She tripped into Ward 1, saw the empty bed, and then went upstairs to the Intensive Care Unit. However, this time, Barbara warned her that I was very, very tired. Doreen was accompanied that day by Dennis Hyde who has himself been put forward for a heart transplant. (At the time of writing, he hasn't had it yet, I know that.) Anyway, this day they both arrived at the Intensive Care Unit.

Sister Screech came up to Doreen and said: 'Look, Mrs Castle, he's ever so tired. Would you mind keeping the visit short?' She and Dennis came over to talk to me, but I didn't join in their conversation much. Doreen said to me: 'Love, would you like me to go home? Is it all a bit much for you?' I didn't want to say so but I had to: 'Yes, love, if you don't mind, could you leave it out?' I think that was the first time I saw Doreen walk out of a hospital crying.

I can't remember for how long I was in the Unit at that time because I lost count of the days with sleeping all the time. I do remember waking up and talking to a young coloured girl in the next bed—that poor unfortunate had been stabbed several times and was in a really critical condition. I'm glad to say that she pulled through. Anyway, there came the inevitable transfer back to Ward 1—bed 11 again as per usual— where the next highlights of my existence were doctors' rounds again, with the Professor and Broughie. As usual the Professor's sense of humour came to the fore and, knowing that I definitely had *not* been told, said to Broughie: 'I say, Dr Brough, have you told Mr Castle that he has now got gout?' 'Gout? Me? Get orf, that's an old man's complaint,' I exclaimed. 'Well, yes, unfortunately you have digitalis intoxication.' (I think that's what he called it.) Well, from the other patients, and of course from Martin and Lodder, I took a lot of stick. From then on, whenever food came round, they would pinch it off my plate, leaving me tiny amounts saying it was far, far too rich for me and it would only aggravate my gout!

One day, Broughie asked me what type of accommodation I was living in. I told him I lived in a Council flat where there were plenty of stairs. Far too many. He asked me how I managed them. I explained that as far as possible I tried to avoid using them, but if I had to it was one stair at a time, sitting down, and it took me about half an hour to do one flight. Broughie wrote to the Council saying, 'this man must have ground floor accommodation—he cannot use stairs'. I received a letter from the Council, which I still treasure to this day. It started out, 'Dear Sir, You are not ill enough . . .' Apparently I fell between categories and I wasn't considered ill enough to warrant ground floor accommodation. The marvellous part was that, the day after my transplant at Papworth (much later on) the Council official got hold of Doreen actually at the hospital and said not '*can* we' but 'we are *going* to rehouse you' which was a bit of a laugh when I didn't have to bother about stairs any more.

3

Hyde Park Corner

Nothing untoward happened to me for a short period, but then I was back in the Unit again. I don't remember exactly what went wrong, but as I said, I was back again. When the night staff came on, I was assigned a temporary nurse—an agency nurse. Now this girl, although she was white, appeared to have an over-exaggerated Indian caste mark on her forehead. She also didn't have a stitch of clothing on underneath her uniform, and she just seemed to act in a peculiar way right from the start. Immediately, the Night Sister had her eagle eye on her. Well, instead of attending to me as she should have done, this nurse was more intent in talking about the heavy-handedness of the government towards all the hippies travelling around Northern India and about their hardships—which wasn't of much interest to me in my state—and all the while she was telling me this, she was setting up a drip bottle. All the other nurses, realising that she was a bit strange, were giving her surreptitious glances whilst attending to their own patients and they whispered amongst themselves when they had the chance. Then my nurse decided she would make me a cup of tea.

In her absence I looked up and, to my horror, she had set the drip at a very fast rate and the solution was now running out like Niagara Falls. I called to the other nurses. 'Now look girls,' I said, 'this ain't funny, come and adjust this drip.' But no—they wouldn't dare interfere with another nurse's patient. In the end I tried to adjust my own drip to a slower running level, with the other nurses looking on. I don't blame them really for not wanting to interfere. It was a good thing for the agency nurse that Night Sister had not seen what was going on! Eventually she called the girl to her and tried to put it nicely—'Did you know you had a bit of chalk on your forehead?' she asked. 'Maybe you'd like to go and wash it off.' The girl started giving her a long-winded explanation about caste marks and Indian hardships again but, with that, the Sister whipped her out of the Unit and I have never seen her from that day to this.

I was soon, however, back to my usual berth of bed 11 in Ward 1, and it was at this time that I had my first brush with the junkies in the ward. Bearing in mind I had only just returned from the Intensive Care Unit,

27

I found it a bit off-putting to be woken up in the middle of the night by a junkie fumbling around in my locker, looking for some cigarettes. In actual fact he was harmless but he was making a terrific noise. He had lost his cigarettes but, in his disoriented state, he was looking in other people's lockers. He got me so mad that I remember standing up on my bed, waving a bed bottle above my head, threatening to crash him on the head with it if he came a step nearer. He moved away from me and went off further down the ward.

In the end bed there was a 92-year-old ex-bookmaker. He was fit and athletic for his age—a very well built fellow—and I don't really know what he was in for. The next minute, of course, the junkie was arguing with him, and it came to a big square up. They started to exchange blows and, funnily enough, I'd have put my money on the old bookmaker, who was well and truly holding his own! The staff soon separated them and no harm was done. But my next encounter with a junkie was the main sore point of my lengthy stay in St James's hospital.

It all started when I was sitting in the little end section of the ward, next to the Day Room, and Gossai came out of the television room. He was white as a sheet and shaking. With some difficulty (because he couldn't speak much English and had a speech impediment) he told me that he had been thrown out of the television room. I knew that watching television was his main pastime, and I couldn't make out why he should be thrown out of the television room, or indeed, who had thrown him out. So, I took Gossai back in there and there was this young junkie, with his girlfriend, huddled up in a corner. She had come to give her boyfriend a fix and had chucked Gossai out of the room so she could do it. I went mad! I stuck Gossai in the seat in front of the television. 'Now, Mr Gossai,' I said, 'we two are going to watch this television programme, and I don't think anything will disturb us.' I glared at the two of them in the corner. They knew they had overdone it and bit their tongues. The rest of the day passed uneventfully.

The very next day, there was a repeat performance. Gossai came out of the television room again, white and shaky, immediately followed by this young girl, who went up to Barbara's office, pleading the cause of her poor boyfriend. She said it was high time he had his *allowed* fix as he was getting the jitters. I followed her down and heard her laying down the law to Barbara and the doctors. I then started marking her card for her. I called her everything barring a Christian. Had she wanted to sue me, she could have taken me for every penny that I had. I told her in no uncertain terms that if either she or her no-good boyfriend ever threw Gossai out of the television room again, I personally would throw the worthless boyfriend out and she would rapidly follow him, with a boot straight up her little arse. Of course, Barbara and the doctors loved it! I could say what they couldn't.

However, it wasn't to end there. A day or two later, Gossai again had cause to complain. He pointed to his pocket and eventually we learned that this junkie and another one had cleaned Gossai out of his fags. It was early in the morning, so they had taken his complete supply. All of us patients went straight to the junkies and made them pay for another packet of fags, which we put in Gossai's pocket. We warned them the dire circumstances they would be in if they ever touched Gossai's cigarettes again.

Just after lunch, I woke up in bed and found, much to my surprise, that I couldn't even turn over. The same two junkies were lying each side of me, on top of my bedclothes, pinning me down. They immediately began scrounging for cigarettes. Luckily I saw a nurse close by. 'Do me a favour, Nurse,' I called, 'get these two clowns off my back.' She took one look, grabbed the junkies and took them away. By now I had had quite enough of them. I demanded to be moved out of Ward 1. I stuck to my guns and said as long as the junkies were there, I wanted to be moved.

I am in no position to criticise junkies, possibly the best thing I could do is to try to understand their position a little better, but I strongly condemn their being put into the general wards of hospitals if they upset sick patients. You can't blame the police, though, for dumping these junkies on hospital doorsteps as they have their job to do and you can't blame the hospitals for having to take them in, after all they *are* sick people, but surely there could be more special units set up to receive them? I'm afraid after the last incident I felt the best place for them was the Council rubbish tip. (This was my personal opinion.)

It was at this time that I met three marvellous fellows, but I must give you the background story about how a big general ward in a hospital operates, before I introduce them to you.

One of the big main wards always has to serve as the intake ward for a certain period. This means that it will have to cope with a big influx of emergency patients being admitted. The nursing staff concerned, therefore, know that they are going to be in for a very busy time especially when the weekend approaches. Quite naturally, the doctors have to use the judgement of Solomon to try to get the wards as empty as possible by sending home those patients who are well on the road to recovery. The nurses, for their part, have to keep juggling the beds about, according to the pecking order—the degree of illness of the patient. Therefore it is not uncommon for a patient to wake up half way through the night to find that his bed has been shifted about and put into a different position in the ward—the nurses literally have to play draughts with the beds.

Ward 1 was intake ward for this particular weekend. Barbara came up to us lads at the end of the ward and warned us that the staff were going to have a pretty hectic time that night and asked if any of us would like to move to the far end of the ward so they could contain the hullabaloo up the other end. Several of the fellows agreed and Barbara said: 'Keith, your breathing isn't too bad at the moment, why don't you go down there too? You could get a better night's sleep. I know there's not an oxygen line on the other side of the barrier, but we could quickly fix you up with a bottle if necessary.'

Subsequently, during the afternoon, we were all settled in at the other end of the ward, and that was when I met John, who was a bus driver, Bob, who tacked up plasterboard on to ceilings, and Harry, who was an income tax fiddler checker upper on! John's job as a bus driver needs no introduction at all, but Harry's job was quite interesting. He used to lead 'flying squads' on his territory of south-east London, from London to the coast, checking up on income tax dodgers, but Bob's story is something worth telling.

Strictly speaking, he shouldn't have been in our ward at all as he had broken a bone in his foot, when some scaffolding collapsed as he was tacking up plasterboard. He should really have been in an orthopaedic ward. Bob was really down in the dumps. At the age of 72 this was the first time he had ever been in hospital in his life. Indeed, it was the first time in his life that he had ever had anything wrong with him. Unfortunately, he had also lost his wife about two weeks earlier. His admittance routine to the hospital didn't help matters. Apparently, following his accident at work, he was brought to the hospital and wheeled to the reception desk. The young clerk filled out his forms and, after asking for his name, age and address etc, she asked Bob for the name of his GP. Bob said he didn't know. 'You must know,' said the girl. 'No I don't,' said Bob, 'you see I've never been to a doctor in my life.' The girl repeated that he *must* have a GP. 'I remember shortly after the war,' continued Bob, 'when the country nationalised the health service or something, my missus signed me up with a chap in Mitcham but he died about 20 years ago.' The young girl tried a different tack. 'When you've been ill in the past, which doctor did you see?' Bob patiently explained that he had never been ill nor seen a doctor. The girl was amazed. 'At 72, never been ill and never seen a doctor,' she exclaimed, 'you must be unique!'

Poor old Bob, not understanding the word 'unique', turned to her and said: 'You saucy young cow—who are you calling unique?' Subsequent enquiries showed that Bob, who had been self-employed all his life, had been paying his full share of income tax and contributions through his accountant. He had never had a rebate and had never been notified about retirement when he was 65.

Well, our little group assembled down the end of the ward and started playing solo. You have all heard of Frank Sinatra's song *The Longest Running Crap Game in the West*? Well, ours was the longest running solo game in the history of the National Health Service! We played it in the majority of wards in St James's Hospital, in St George's Hospital and even in the Barrier Room at Papworth Hospital. Out of the four of us, if there was one in hospital and the other three were out-patients then these three would come in as visitors, and out would come the cards. Most times this wouldn't have mattered, but there was one episode where Harry was back in St James's—although not in Ward 1—and the other three of us went in to see him. Well, it wasn't long before the cards came out and we were all round Harry's bed playing solo.

Harry didn't feel too good, and the nurse went and got him some oxygen. Whilst she was screwing the mask on to the bottle, I (as I was feeling absolutely terrible at the time) jokingly, but half-seriously, said to her: 'I could do with some of that as well, nurse.' She thought I was trying to be funny, and snapped my head off, and it wasn't until later on that she realised that I was, in fact, in a very bad way. Having watched me closely she told the Ward Sister about my condition. Anyhow, soon after that, the card school broke up. We said goodnight to Harry and left.

As soon as we had gone, the Sister went to Harry and said: 'Look here, whenever your friends visit you again, you are *not* to play cards because you get yourself all excited and put your blood pressure right up, and don't you *ever* let that friend of yours, who is so short of breath, come in this ward without giving me ample notice, I want to keep my eye on him. Now, what is the score with him, and how bad is he?'

Of course, Harry told her that I was an 'in-and-out patient' of Ward 1, and had I been in dire trouble, I would have had the sense to ask her to get me down to that ward quickly. That made Sister even more worried, so she went down to Ward 1 and had a chat with Barbara. Barbara put her in the picture and, after that, whenever we visited Harry, the Sister didn't mind because she knew the situation—but her eagle eye was well and truly on me during the whole period of my visits there.

There then followed an incident, which some people would say was fate, destiny, the largest stroke of luck that anybody was to have in life, etc . . . but it was the one incident that was to lead me directly on the path to Papworth Hospital. I was attending the Out-patients at St James's at that time, and I was with a registrar with whom I had never had much contact. This registrar gave me a real bolt out of the blue. 'Mr Castle,' she said, 'there's no need for you to come to any more clinics here, just go home, draw your pills from your local GP and that will be good enough.'

Well, when I got home to Doreen, I was laughing. 'That's it,' I said, 'she's signed my death warrant now—I've been chucked out of St James's and that's all there is to it!' 'What do you mean, chucked out of St James's?' answered Doreen. 'Just what I told you,' I replied, 'I ain't got to go back there any more—she's just sent me home to die.' This, let's face it, was the truth.

In the post the next morning, I received an Out-patients appointment for the following week. I duly attended. The registrar looked up at me in surprise, saying: 'I thought I signed you off last week?' 'So you did, but look, this came in the post.' I showed her the appointment booking. She said there must have been some sort of mistake. 'Well,' I said, 'I'm glad there was a mistake, 'cos I feel so awful I would have come in anyway.' So she asked me to strip off, get on the couch, so that she could have a look at me. After she had given me an examination, she said, very seriously: 'Look, if you'll promise to give up smoking, I'll arrange for you to see the cardiologist at St George's Hospital. But, you've got to promise me to give up smoking and not waste their time.'

I knew that was a bit of bluster on her part to keep me on my toes, because with the state of my breathing at that time, I could no more have smoked a cigarette than have flown to the moon. Anyhow, if she suggested a visit to the cardiologist at St George's—who was I to argue? All in all, it was far better than being chucked out of hospital altogether.

St George's hospital was in a transitional stage at that time. They were shifting it from its traditional site at Hyde Park Corner, to the suburbs of Tooting and had plans to build around the two existing hospitals there. This changeover period was going to take years. The registrar gave me the choice of going to Tooting or to Hyde Park Corner—whichever was the easiest for me to travel to. I didn't mind which so I said 'Tooting' and that was where the appointment was made.

Eventually, I arrived at Tooting to see this cardiologist. I wondered what sort of a God he was, having been told not to smoke in front of him! I opened the door, and there sat Dr David Redwood.

This is how our first meeting went. (Although I am doing this book from memory, and I may be way out on dates etc, my first conversation with Dr David Redwood I remember—word perfect!) As I walked in, he looked up and said very courteously: 'Good morning Mr Castle!' 'Good morning, Doc,' was my reply. He looked up. 'Oh, do you call every doctor by that name?' 'Only till I know them better,' I quipped, 'and then I tell them the truth!' 'Good!' he said. 'That is the attitude I want you to keep with me. I don't want you to hold anything back—I want you to feel completely at ease, and we'll keep that up for as long as we know each other.' This we have done to this day.

After having examined me thoroughly and having read through all my notes, Dr Redwood arranged for me to go up to Hyde Park Corner to have a catheter test. I didn't realise it at the time, but this was when I was to leave the general wards for good and find myself in the world of cardiology. Having pleasantly discovered that Dr Redwood didn't have three heads and breathe fire, I soon found I was to have my first introduction to Harris Ward, and to Maggie—the Ward Sister.

I'll describe Maggie first, because, of all the medical people I mention in this book, she is the only one who has subsequently left the NHS. (Alma from Papworth, who I talk of later on, is still vaguely connected with it.) Also I intend to talk about Maggie in more detail than anyone else. It is a safe bet to say that every single patient who has been under Maggie's care, holds the view that she must be the world's finest cardiology Ward Sister. Every digression that she let us get away with was all calculated carefully by her as a morale booster. She was neither hard on her nurses nor weak with them. At the beginning of the day's session she would gently explain to them what was expected of each and every one of them, and the nurses would willingly and happily get on with it. She had a similar rapport with the patients. On the odd occasion, when she did have to give a stroppy patient a flea in the ear, there was no holding her back! However, because of the way she ran things, those sort of occasions were very few and far between. Anyway, you will read about Maggie as and when she crops up—but now, we'll get back to Harris Ward.

Harris Ward was 'T'-shaped. The bottom leg of the 'T' was the Men's ward, with only a few beds in it. On the cross-section of the 'T', on the left-hand side and as small as the Men's ward, was the Women's. The right-hand section led into a very long ward called Grosvenor Ward. So Harris Ward was the bottom half of the 'T' and the left-hand top piece. All the patients in Harris Ward were what you could call 'hot potato' heart cases. They were either patients who were very seriously ill or ones who were returning for their second and third heart operations.

The most unfortunate part of St George's, Hyde Park, was the traffic outside. There was only a pavement's width between the densest traffic in the whole of Great Britain and the ward. Consequently, every window had to be tightly double-glazed. The antiquated ventilation system couldn't adequately cope with the air and, in the hot summer seasons, I have known the staff to have borrowed fans from every conceivable place to try to cool the patients down. When you realise that some of these patients had great difficulty in breathing anyway, you will understand how uncomfortable things were. The *only* place where you could have some sort of fresh air was in the toilets—which were only single glazed—so the toilets became the meeting place for all the patients in the ward! Not a very clinical meeting place, I'll agree, but sometimes it was hilariously funny in there.

During my few days in Harris Ward for my catheter and other tests, my breathing was at its worst ever. I was literally paralysed with it. They increased my diuretic tablets to 500 mg a day and I believe, for one short period, I was on 750 mg a day, but 500 from then on seemed to be my standard dose, which was rather a lot.

A few days after my discharge from St George's, I was on my way to St James's as an out-patient to the dental registrar. I had some loose teeth in the bottom of my mouth as the result of doing a stupid thing. Before my first heart attack, I had tried to pull off the rubber covering from some electric leading with my teeth. Unfortunately, I got the copper wire hooked around my teeth and loosened them. They had been troubling me ever since but, because of my heart condition, the dental registrar at St James's wouldn't touch them. He said Professor Pilkington had advised that it would be far too dangerous (possibly I wouldn't survive the necessary treatment). I was always trying to gee them up into taking these teeth out, but they would have none of it and it became a nice, long-running battle.

Anyway, as I was saying, I was on my way to the dental clinic when, all of a sudden, my left leg went dead. It just stiffened up, I could barely move or walk. Therefore, instead of getting myself to the dental surgery, I carried on to the heart clinic. I told the Sister on duty what had happened and she put me straight into a cubicle. Both registrars who were on duty at the time (Doctors Cochram and Johnston) came in to see me. They gave my leg a quick checkover, and decided I had either had an embolism or a thrombosis as the result of the catheter test. It's unfortunate, but these things must happen just now and again, particularly for someone like me with a long relationship with the Health Service. Still, ever since, I have had trouble with this leg and it does play me up when I walk. It claudicates when I first set off but, after I have been walking a little while, the feeling goes off. I'll probably have this trouble for years to come.

The familiar routine then followed. I was admitted straight away into Ward 1, without going home, bed 11 again, and Doreen soon came in with my gear. The next few days were a bit of a worrying period for Professor Pilkington in case I had a stroke, or anything like that, but eventually he was satisfied that I would be all right. It was soon after this that one of the registrars put it to me that they would like to transfer me permanently to St George's Hospital. I enquired whether or not that would entail any surgery and I was given the same answer which I had received many times—no, I wasn't going to be operated on, there was nothing that could be done for me. So, to me, although I liked St George's Hospital a lot, it was a pointless move. Why change one physician you are quite happy with, for another? They tried to dissuade me from this view, but I stood firm. They reported my feelings to

Professor Pilkington and he agreed with me—if the patient is happy where he is, let him stay there.

There was one occasion, when John, Bob, Harry and myself first met up, when we were sitting around quietly talking when John turned to me and said: 'Hey, Keith, you've been around hospitals a long time now, can you tell me why some of the beds have boards underneath them— you know, like sheets of plywood?' 'Well, actually, John,' I said, 'that's mainly for heart patients. It's in case something goes wrong with you and they need to thump your chest hard—well the board stops you bouncing up and down in the bed whilst they're doing it! There's another thing, John. I don't want to worry you, but I've noticed one thing. I had my second heart attack exactly seven days after my first one, and two or three of my contemporaries have as well. I'm not saying that that is the usual thing—but I've seen it happen so much in my time. Why don't *you* take it easy today—because today is *your* seventh day!'

We all laughed about this, but all day long John 'geed' me up a bit by saying he was taking things very steady! Towards the end of the day he said: 'So much for your theory about a second attack on the seventh day—nothing's happened to me.' But just then, Henry (one of the nurses) walked down the ward pushing a big trolley, with two of these big plywood boards on it. He immediately put one of these underneath John's mattress. We all burst out laughing but this laughter doubled when he put the other one underneath *my* bed!

That was the first time that John really accepted that he had a bad heart because he carried rather a lot of excess weight. However, after subsequent tests over the following months, the outlook became rosier and rosier for John, but he did have to look for another job as obviously he couldn't continue to be a bus driver. He wanted to get a job as a trainee pub manager. He arranged to see Dr Cochram, not in his clinic, but privately, just to talk about it and ask his opinion. Cochram said it would be no good if John had, physically, to hump barrels about, etc, so John promised to get a good cellar man. The only other problem was the question of John bending his right elbow. He said that if John could control what he drank there was no reason why he could not pursue this line of business. Anyway, John did try the pub game, but in the end he had to give it up. Before he did, Bob, Harry and myself decided to go and visit him at North Harrow when we were again out-patients.

We had our usual good get-together. We sat round the table, laughing and joking, but this was another occasion when I possibly had another heart attack. I did feel rough! Not wanting to spoil the fun I popped a couple of pills in my mouth. I never did really suffer from angina, but I always had tablets around me, just in case something happened. John saw me do this, but didn't say a word to the others until the meeting was just breaking up, when he had a go at me. 'Look at this berk here,' he said to the others, 'fancy not letting on he's had an attack. I saw you popping pills into your mouth!' They all told me off, but they knew I would have mentioned it to them had things got out of hand.

After this, we all piled in the car to go home. When we were all in, Bob decided to light up the biggest cigar I have ever seen in my life. It was horrible—it was literally choking me. Once again, not wishing to spoil the fun, I stuck it out. As soon as the car stopped outside my place, I said goodnight hurriedly and bowled straight indoors, where I was promptly very sick!

Nothing much happened from that period until Christmas 1978— apart from one funny incident with Dr Wells! At this stage, I was such a physical wreck that I was impotent as well as everything else. So one day, I turned to Wellsie and said: 'Now look, let's review my position. I can't smoke because I can't breathe. I can't have a drink because it makes me vomit and the only thing I can raise is a smile! I can't even climb up the stairs to chuck myself off the roof! Will I ever be able to get at least *one* of those three deadly sins back again?' Wellsie replied: 'Well, at this stage, your breathing's bad, so I can't see what we can do about smoking; your duodenal ulcer is bad, so I can't see what we can do about drinking . . .' 'Right,' I said, 'that only leaves one thing left. Will I ever be like one of those little rabbits on Salisbury Plain and breed like a lunatic?' Wellsie smiled. 'To tell the truth, I didn't know you were impotent,' he replied, 'it must be all your pills—I'll see if I can get them adjusted.'

I knew he was only fobbing me off, but I let it go for a few days. Then I jokingly asked him about it again. Wellsie looked me straight in the eye and, with an old fashioned look, put his left hand across his right upper arm, bringing the lower arm up in the time-honoured symbol and said: 'Look—you've got two choices—you can either have this and die, or go without it and live.' What could I say after that? However if I am going to be told things, then that's the way I'd prefer to be told—no old fashioned pronouncements, but a doctor being entirely natural with you.

During Christmas 1978, we were at home. All the kids came to spend the holiday with us and it was the usual type of family Christmas. Doreen and I visited Sister Screech in the ICU. Doreen had made some table decorations and taken them into the Unit. Of course, they couldn't be put in the Unit itself, so we left them scattered around the big Christmas tree just outside, and then went down to see Barbara with more decorations. Altogether, it was a nice, enjoyable little Christmas. I'm glad it was because, shortly after this, I was faced with the drumming out ceremony from St James's Hospital.

I was in the clinic one day, when Dr Johnston said: 'Fair do's, from now on you are a St George's patient.' I said: 'What do you mean?' He replied: 'Well, whether you like it or not, you are no longer a patient at St James's. I have transferred you to St George's.' I had the hump. I *really* had the hump over it. However, it was no good and that was that. Still, as I went out of the door I said to him: 'Well, you've got rid of me, but I'll tell you—I'll be back!'

So, from then on I was to attend Out-patients at St George's. This was a unique experience for any heart patient, because the heart clinic was housed in the depths of St George's and at that hospital, every little bit of it seemed to be built on a different level from the next one. It was all split level with lots of ramps from one floor to another. The Cardiac Clinic consisted of a corridor which sloped downward, with chairs on each side. The out-patients sat here and, to be honest, it was just like sitting in a rather long bus.

My routine followed its usual course . . . Out-patients at Hyde Park Corner, home again, lounging about, vomiting, etc, etc, but all the while trying to get on with a bit of painting, which was my passionate hobby. Doreen and I enjoyed this quiet life that we were able to lead. Doreen's main hobby was flower arranging—every Friday night, at the local Institute. I could attend as many art classes as I chose to at the Institute, but unfortunately I began to go less and less, for the simple reason that the classes were held on the 8th floor, and the stairs were too much for me. Mind you, the tutor in charge, to help me out, had placed chairs at various strategic points on the staircase landings, so that I could have a rest and take all the time in the world to reach the class. However, unfortunately for me, the area Fire Officer inspected the place and pointed out that the chairs were blocking fire exits, so they had to be removed. Consequently, I could no longer make the stairs.

4

Papworth—where's that?

One day, I felt rough. Doreen and I debated whether I should go to the hospital or not. I didn't like being a time-waster and, let's be fair, if I had gone to the hospital every time I felt rough, I'd never have left the place! As the day went on, I felt worse, and worse. Towards late afternoon, things were really bad so Doreen said: 'Come on, you're definitely going to the hospital.' She didn't quite know which one of the two St Georges to telephone—Hyde Park Corner or Tooting. She tried Tooting but, as I said, it was in the middle of the big changeover, and Doreen couldn't get any sense out of anyone there. I expect it was because poor Doreen was in a bit of a state at this moment. Nevertheless, she then rang Hyde Park Corner. Nick, the registrar on duty, told her: 'Look, Mrs Castle, although he is not on my list, I know your husband's case history quite well. From what you tell me, I shall admit him, but I'm not sure which ward he will be admitted to. Could you ring back in five minutes' time so that I can give you the answer and you can bring him straight to the ward?'

Five minutes elapsed and Doreen rang again. 'OK, Mrs Castle, bring him in to Drummond Ward,' Nick told her. 'Get a cab and bring him straight in. If you haven't got the cash for a cab, don't worry at all—we'll pay the fare at this end, and don't go through all the formalities downstairs, just bring him directly to Drummond Ward.'

We then had the job of trying to get a cab. As usual, whenever you want one in emergency, you can't find one! We didn't consider an ambulance because, although an ambulance would have taken me to St George's, Tooting, because of zonal differences they could not cross the river to take me to the twin hospital, St George's at Hyde Park Corner. A strange anomaly, but I was stuck with it.

After a while we managed to find one. The cabbie looked down his nose at me as I was in my dressing gown and slippers! He most probably didn't want anything going wrong in his cab whilst we were en route! Anyhow, we arrived at St George's. It was now well into the evening when I was admitted to Drummond Ward and Nick examined me and then said: 'I won't pull any punches, you're in chronic heart failure so I have a strong feeling that you are going to be remaining here

38

for some time.' He was right! Doreen went home and I was settled down in the ward.

By now, it was time for all the patients to go to sleep. They fixed me up with two 'IVAC' machines. These are automatic drug dispensing machines, like a glorified drip. The only trouble is that, if the machine should happen to go wrong and the drugs are not dispensed in the minute volumes as they should be, an alarm buzzer goes off. For the whole of that night, the buzzer on one of my two machines was going off all the time. The rest of the poor patients in the ward were moaning and groaning and yelling out, but there was nothing to be done about it and the nurses spent all their time trying to rectify the matter. It was just one of those things. I think everybody from the Sister to the nurses and the patients were so, so glad when they transferred me from Drummond Ward to the ward in which they wanted to get me in the first place, Harris Ward.

After I had settled in there, Dr Redwood came around and introduced me to Dr Bill Ginks, the Senior Registrar Cardiologist there. From then on I was Bill's patient and his worry, and I am glad to say I was, because what Bill did for me was absolutely unbelievable. But for Bill, it would have been just one long uphill struggle without any improvements—just setback after setback after setback. At least that's how it appeared to me, but in fact Bill's greatest triumph was just keeping me alive. More especially he kept me alive and got me into a suitable condition to get up to Papworth and face all that happened to me up there.

For weeks and weeks it was try this, try that and try the other, to get some improvement in my condition. All the time we were struggling. I don't know whether it was Bill's decision to get me to Papworth during this period or not, however Papworth comes later in my story.

To settle down in Harris Ward was no great hardship for me, I was so used to the hospital routine. To tell the truth, apart from the physical sight of them, you would not have realised that the other patients were drastically ill heart patients. It was almost as if they had got a collection of the greatest comedians in the country and assembled them in Harris Ward. We literally never stopped laughing! The jokes and situation comedies were just going on all the time. It was all absolutely spontaneous and the greatest tonic any patient could ever have.

My bed was slightly apart from the others. I believe it was raised on one step and was slightly forward so that it projected itself into the ward. With the curtains going round the top of it, it took little imagination to see a four-poster bed—and it quickly was dubbed 'Castle's Corner'. However, the ward was so small that, even in casual conversation, you could be heard from one end of it to the other, so I wasn't isolated.

By then, my legs and ankles were well and truly bloated and my liquid intake was being reduced daily, down to its eventual level of *only* 600 cc a day. In addition I was still on 500 mg of diuretics per day and the weather also was boiling hot so I rapidly got into a very sorry state with a terrific thirst and cracked lips. My day's liquid intake therefore called for the application of higher mathematics. Should I either have three small cups of tea at 180 cc a throw, and leave a little drop for soup, should I forego soup, or what? In the end I chose to have half cups of tea so that I could spread them out throughout the day. I also assumed that with half cups of tea there might be a tendency for the orderly to be a big generous in his pouring! Mind you, I could have had some Guinness, which St George's allowed its patients in order to build them up, but, as I say, in the end it was half cups of tea which I chose.

The nurses were very kind—because the ward was so stuffy in the hot weather, they let me suck a small ice cube sometimes. This helped a lot. Doreen also brought in some ice lollies and the nurses put these in the fridge and occasionally let me have a suck of one, so I did get by all right, although it wasn't very pleasant. At least this stopped my lips from cracking too badly.

I always had to have some ice standing by though, because I needed to bite on it when I was having one particular drug. I won't name the drug in case those patients on it now get the wrong end of the stick about it, but I had to take it intravenously in large doses and I don't think that anything I have ever had in hospital has been so painful. It was excruciating! It was far worse than a drug I subsequently went on at Papworth, where they quickly discontinued using it. It wasn't helped by the fact that nurse Celia, lovely girl though she was, had a bit of muscle on her and she could pump this drug in with all the force of a fire hose. Although I have a fairly high pain threshold, I just couldn't have faced it again and again had I not had that ice to bite on. The worst thing was, I had to have *two* injections and I'll never forget the dreadful feeling of waiting for the second needle. I don't think I ever did chicken out of having it. Dear Celia, she has now moved on to John Radcliffe Hospital at Oxford, or she had the last time I heard of her, and I often wonder how many patients down there are getting the same type of treatment from her!

As you can see, at this time ice played a big part in my life, but it became more and more difficult to store it in the ward fridge, all because of a patient whom we had named Tom Sawyer. His real name was Roland. Roland had a job which involved designing fermentation tanks for a big brewery concern. As his brewery bought up smaller breweries throughout the country, Roland's job was to go to them, update and re-design their fermentation tanks and get a Danish firm in to build them. He saw to the whole operation, from start to finish.

Whenever visitors from these breweries came down to London, they always brought him cans of beer. All I could say was that Roland must have designed a lot of fermentation tanks in his time and there were certainly a lot of generous brewery managers travelling to London. Soon the beer filled all the fridges, to the total exclusion of drugs, my ice—the lot. Although the fridges were overflowing with beer, no one took advantage of this, because we were all too ill to drink the stuff.

By now, I had got to know a fellow patient—Percy Ayres—quite well. Percy and I were to tread similar paths in the future, right up to Papworth and beyond. Percy will forgive me for saying so, but he had an *evil* sense of humour! I could tell you stories from now to kingdom come about Percy, and never run out!

My first introduction to his humour came via George, another patient in the ward. George was happily telling us a story about his holidays in Majorca at one of the hotels there. Percy pricked up his ears when George came out with the profound statement that 'a packet of fags and a pint of beer only cost you a few potatoes'. Percy knew he had a fall guy from then on. He engaged George in earnest conversation, wanting to find out more about this holiday and what else you could buy for a few potatoes. Before long, George was passing round photographs of the holiday and Percy soon found one photograph of George sitting in a chair with two chorus girls on his lap. He thought that George might have done a bit of pub singing in his time. Percy turned to George and said: 'Your face is very familiar to me, have you been an entertainer in your time?' Well, George, who had not performed anywhere, other than in the local boozer, replied: 'Yes, of course, I used to do quite a lot of singing and entertaining.' He began to preen himself. 'I thought so,' answered Percy, 'but you were only a singer, weren't you? You couldn't do one of those one-man band acts.' 'Well,' said George, 'I certainly never did anything like that, but I definitely could.' 'Never in a million years,' said Percy, with a twinkle in his eye. With that, George, in the middle of a cardiac ward, jumped up on to his bed and started gyrating, just as a one-man band would have done. Unfortunately, as he reached the peak of his performance, he got carried away and fell off the bed! We thought no more about it that night, but retribution came the following morning, when it was discovered that George had broken his arm. So Maggie quickly put a stop to that sort of thing and public entertainments ceased in the ward from then on.

On another occasion, a chap called Bert was going down for his heart operation and Percy was going down for a catheter investigation, which meant that they both had to go into the toilets and shave off. Young Jenny, the nurse, gave them a razor apiece. After they had shaved, Percy turned to Bert and said: 'Hey, these razors are still sharp—let's have a face shave whilst we are about it. It will save going back up to the ward for our own toilet gear.' Just as they had got the lather around their faces, Jenny happened to walk into the bathroom. The look of horror on her face was a sight to see when she saw the lather around their faces instead of their nether regions. It was marvellous to watch.

'No, no!' she cried, 'you're not supposed to shave *there*.' Percy immediately began to take the mickey. 'What do you mean, love,' he asked, 'you gave us razors to shave with, and that's what we are doing!' 'No, no,' repeated Jenny, 'you're not supposed to be shaving your *faces*—you're meant to be shaving elsewhere, if you know what I mean?' Percy laughed, 'Well, if that's all you're worried about, love,' he said, and proceeded to drop his trousers to show he had already done it! This was followed by a rather ribald remark which was shouted out at Jenny who immediately fled!

Among other things that I was taking at this time, during Dr Ginks's struggle to help me, was an experimental paste and I shall never shake off the feeling that this paste, at a later stage, actually saved my life. It was a paste designed for the exclusive use of angina sufferers. Usually you had to wait until you suffered an angina attack and then you put a pill under your tongue. The theory behind this paste was that it was spread in small measured amounts across your body and then covered with some greaseproof paper. The slow absorption of it would keep the arteries open all the time.

Now, although angina itself wasn't one of my problems, it was always a risk. I remember Professor Pilkington, throughout my lengthy dealings with him, putting his arm around my shoulder whilst he talked to me, but all the time he put his thumb on my Venus point to see what the pressure was. It was always extremely high. Bill Ginks, however, simply used the paste on me because I had no blood circulating around my body—my arteries were as flat as a pancake. He used it merely to keep my veins and arteries open. I swear to this day that, after my heart transplant at Papworth, this paste, having done such a good job in keeping these vessels open, allowed the blood to run round freely from my new healthy heart—without exploding the whole arterial system. It may be an uneducated opinion, but I shall never be shaken from it.

Visiting me in Harris Ward in St George's was becoming a bit of a strain for Doreen because it wasn't so easy to get to as St James's had been. (To reach St James's from our house was easy because there was virtually a door-to-door bus service, also the visiting hours were very free and easy.) At Harris Ward, there were only two visiting times per day, one in the afternoon and one in the evening. Doreen used to come in during the afternoon, but on the return journey there was always that rush through the dense rush hour traffic round Hyde Park Corner back to Battersea. I used to encourage her to have the odd day off, but she wouldn't have it and always came in every single day. But it was a strain on her. She had to make her visits in the afternoon because of our son, Kevin, and even then she had to leave him for some time when he came out of school. She couldn't possibly bring him straight from school, after a quick meal, through all that Hyde Park Corner traffic to visit me in the evening—that would have been just too much for him. So the afternoon visit was the lesser of two evils for Doreen. Mind you, I was lucky that she was able to come every day. Many patients lived a long way away and therefore only had visitors at weekends. One poor chap came from the Channel Islands, so he had no visitors at all.

Thursdays, as was the case for most hospitals in the country, was discussion day for all the doctors. That was the day on which they would meet to go over the patients' notes. The routine with our cardiologists was that they would walk through Harris Ward, through the toilets at the back, up an iron staircase and into a room, which was their meeting place. Dr Leatham was in charge (I don't think I saw him to actually talk to until I had returned from Papworth) but every Thursday, he was kept fully notified of my condition by Bill and Dr Redwood. I can assure any patient here and now that, if you think you are being ignored by the top brass whilst you are in hospital, you are wrong. They are always kept fully up to date about your condition and it's usually on Thursdays when they make all the big decisions.

We used to watch Maggie intently each Thursday, as she made her way through the loos, up the spiral staircase to the room above, carrying a tray of tea and biscuits. We kept hoping that she would have to put the tray down as she passed through one day, in order to answer the 'phone or something, so that out of sheer devilment we would be able to spike the doctors' tea (with the venue being the loos and as we were all on diuretics, the reasons for wishing to spike the doctors' tea are obvious!)

I can remember one day, I had been fast asleep in my bed, when I woke up and couldn't really believe what I was looking at opposite me. I got out of bed and put on my slippers and went down the other end of the ward to Percy. 'I can't believe what I'm seeing,' I told him, 'come up the other end of the ward and confirm it for me.' Percy, sensing that something was in the wind, trotted after me.

What caused all the amusement was a patient called Paddy. He was standing on the platform scales, trying to weigh himself. However hard he tried, he couldn't make the scales tell his correct weight. This was obvious to us onlookers because, lying across the platform of the scales were the big, thick, X-ray cables, adding to his weight. 'What on earth are you playing at, Paddy?' we asked. 'I've been trying to weigh myself for ages,' he answered, 'but these scales are wrong!' We patiently told him to look down at his feet. He still couldn't get it. 'What about those cables?' we said. 'Can't you see that the weight of those is adding to the weight of your body?' 'You're right, boys,' he cried and, with that, he bent down, picked up the cables and, still holding them in his hands, he started to weigh himself again! 'By Jees! That's better,' he said. I don't think the person who invented Irish jokes could beat this true story!

Sometimes, when I had spells of being too rough to get out of bed, Maggie would say to me: 'If you want a cigarette, why don't you draw your curtains and have a quiet puff?' As my bed stood slightly apart from all the others, I could pull the curtains right round it. I have never been a believer in smoking in a ward where there are patients with breathing troubles—I've been on the receiving end of that many times. I also didn't smoke very much at that time anyway, although a cigarette now and again was very nice. So, with Maggie's help, I would draw my curtains, take in a wash bowl to let the others think that that's what I was doing, and have a quiet drag. In order to avoid the smoke going all over the ward, I took what I thought were good precautions and exhaled through a wet flannel.

Celia, who was always on the ball, often spotted the smoke coming up over the top of my curtains and would yell out: 'Keith! Is that smoke coming out from your cubicle?' 'No, no, Celia,' I would reply, 'It's just steam from me washbowl!' The trick of blowing through the flannel must have worked because, whenever she poked her head through the curtains, she did not pursue the matter further. I always got away with it and Maggie and I used to have a good laugh about it! That was the beauty of Maggie. She knew when she could bend a rule, she knew when she could let *us* do so, too. It wasn't habitual, but was always at an appropriate time, in order to give her patient a little pick-up. The old saying that rules are meant to be broken does sometimes apply. Another thing that Maggie would do was to slip me a glass of sherry now and again—not because I was despondent or anything, I can never remember being despondent—no, it was just to give her patient a little pleasure in life.

I think that it was about this time that Bill decided to put me forward for a possible heart transplant. I was still suffering with my teeth. Those loose teeth which they were unable to take out were now quite bad and, of course, any prospective heart transplant patient had to have the matter put right because of infection after the operation. Even a slightly receding gum is a source of infection, but bad teeth have definitely to come out. Anyway, Maggie had a word with me about my teeth and, in no time at all, I was down in Dentistry having them removed. In retrospect, I feel sure a decision regarding transplantation must have been made by then. I don't know whether or not Maggie had jumped the gun, but when Bill heard that I had been down to have my teeth out he went, as far as he ever did, stark staring mad! He tore a real strip off Maggie! I don't suppose I will ever know exactly when the decision was made about my transplant. At that time I hadn't been told about it and certainly hadn't been accepted for it. Anyway, I was pleased. I had had those wretched teeth out and it certainly saved any worries as far as they were concerned when I eventually did get to Papworth.

I remember this period as being very pleasant. I was tired and spent a great deal of my time on my bed sleeping. It was a nice sort of tiredness, with absolutely no worries at all—it was almost ecstatic. Speaking of ecstasy, the great kick for me at this period was bathing my feet. You couldn't compare St Tropez, Copacabana or any of the world's exotic beaches with a paddle in the Harris Ward at that time! Maggie would run a cold bath and add lots of salt to it. Then I would just sit for hours on the edge of the bath dangling my red hot, bloated, old legs in the saline solution to cool them off.

Now I come to think of it, Maggie must have a bath fetish—many stories about her concern baths! On one occasion there was a poor old patient called Les who was really too ill and too fat to have a bath. However, he insisted and the upshot was that he became well and truly jammed in. All the nurses tried to get him out, but to no avail. If they'd taken our advice in the first place, and tied a rope round Les's neck for everyone to pull together, then Maggie would not have needed to take off her tights, hitch up her kilt and get into the bath behind Les and, from a very undignified position, give one almighty heave and pop Les out like a cork! We claimed that for ages afterwards she had a wistful look in her eye—not surprising, only she knew what parts she touched under water to obtain initial lift off!

One day, I was woken from one of my pleasant sleeps by a great commotion going on at the other end of the ward. Apparently, Percy had been having an academic argument with a chap and was losing badly, so once again he resorted to his wicked sense of humour. He was arguing with a Jewish bloke—a really nice, likeable, harmless chappie. 'Anyway, I don't know why you're wasting your time arguing with me over things at all,' said Percy. 'Do you realise that tomorrow you are going to have a pig's valve stuck in your heart!' The poor chap hadn't thought of a pig's valve before and kosher pigs were hardly flooding the market! He called for Maggie and she in turn called Bill. They could not pacify the poor fellow and I never did find out what sort of valve he eventually received. Anyhow, for a while the ward was in total uproar, with Percy grinning all over his face—he'd scored at last!

I then ran into another period when I was vomiting continuously. Basically, I think it was because I was on some Clofibrate capsules to clear the excessive cholesterol in my body as I had quite a big build-up of cholesterol by then. These capsules seemed to aggravate my ulcer, hence the vomiting. I thought I had got used to all hospital routines and had lost all sense of shyness—many's the time that nurses had to help me in and out of baths; I wasn't worried about that, but the vomiting was always a source of great embarrassment to me. I hated the thought of the nurses having to clear up after me.

On one occasion, Maggie had allowed me to go down for a bath. Shortly before this, I had eaten some juicy black grapes. I had a lovely bath and felt fine. However, whilst I was bending over to clean the bath afterwards—and of course I shouldn't have been doing that—I started to vomit and up came all the grapes! I sat on the chair for a few minutes until I gathered enough strength to leave the bathroom and ask one of the other patients to ask a nurse to pop into the bathroom when she was free. It was now visiting time. I returned to the job of trying to clean up the bath. When Jenny arrived she was horrified when she saw me and told me to go back to bed. 'No, love,' I said, 'it's not on for you to clear that up after me.' But it was no good. Jenny *insisted* on taking me back to my bed before she returned to clear up the ghastly mess. The next minute, she came rushing back to me. 'Keith, what on earth have you been eating?' she asked, looking worried. She had seen all the black grape skins and had mistaken them for blood clots! She was so relieved when I told her I had just had some grapes. But I hated the girls having to clear up after me like that—I really did. What with that, and other vomiting episodes, I was so glad when Dr Redwood took me off those awful capsules. I was particularly pleased I was off them when I had possibly the greatest treat ever during my stay in Harris Ward.

Percy had been allowed home for a time. Unfortunately, par for the course, he was soon back—but, in the meantime he had caught two beautiful eels and made up two huge cartons of jellied eels. He brought these in for me as a treat. We put them in the fridge, and that night I said to John, the charge nurse: 'Do you like jellied eels?' John replied that he had never tried them so I told him that this was his golden opportunity to find out, provided he brought us plenty of vinegar and pepper. I didn't know whether this was allowed on my diet or not, but I was determined to enjoy my treat. John obliged and, on tasting them, he found to his surprise, but intense pleasure, that he really liked jellied eels. We polished the lot off between us! As I said, it was a wonderful treat and all thanks to Percy for springing that surprise on me.

Later on, although I didn't realise it at the time, I was able to help Percy because both he and I were on some special pills which were flown in for us from America. No one else was on them. Eventually, Percy was getting short of these particular pills and Bill was becoming worried about where to get a supply. Fortunately, in the medicine chest, they found some of these pills which had been allocated to me, but they had been left behind when I went to Papworth, so that prevented Percy from going short.

Life in Harris Ward continued in its inevitable way, with the nurses carrying out their duties quietly and efficiently under Maggie's guidance. The usual jokes were made about me being indestructible. Dr Robertson said that if a bus hit me, they would have to tow the bus away and I would continue on my way with no ill-effects. Percy's sense of humour always helped, and life went on, with a good time being had by all—as far as was possible in the circumstances.

However, events began to speed up for me. I was the subject of a series of tests conducted by Bill, and these tests were due to last about five days, for a couple of hours each day. They largely consisted of pumping phials of ice cold liquid into me and, through the computer, seeing how my heart reacted.

On about the third day, towards the end of the tests, Bill leaned over and asked: 'Keith, when you were in here last year for catheter studies, what was your attitude towards surgery?' 'Bill, you know full well that I have never been allowed to *have* an attitude towards surgery,' I replied, 'I've always been told that I wouldn't survive it, and that there was no operation that *I* could have anyway.' 'Well,' he responded, 'if there was a possible chance, what would be your attitude now?' The penny dropped immediately. Although he hadn't actually used the word 'transplantation', I knew what was in the back of his mind. I was on to it like a hawk. 'What do you mean—explain!' I said. 'Now, don't get carried away,' he answered. 'If I could possibly get you up to Cambridge to see some people up there, would you object if there was the chance of any surgery at the end of it?' I was pretty excited and virtually throttled him! 'As I said—don't get carried away,' he cautioned, 'certain things have to happen, but I can send your clinical papers up there for their opinion, but I cannot convey your personality to them—it's up to you to show them that you are up to it. You must hold your horses for a few days until I can get you more information.'

After that phase of testing, I got back to the ward and immediately telephoned my sister, Joan. I asked her if she could arrange to bump into Doreen when she visited me at about five o'clock that day, making it look like an accident, and pretend she had just come to visit me, too. I explained to Joan that I had something to tell Doreen and I didn't want her to go home on her own afterwards, in case she was upset. Joan readily agreed.

The two of them eventually arrived at my ward. I explained that it had been suggested that there was a slight possibility of me going to Cambridge and that there was a possibility of a heart transplant being done. Doreen took the news in her stride, but my sister didn't, and it was Doreen who had to support *her* home that night!

The occupants of Harris Ward quite typically all started making ribald jokes about heart transplant patients when they heard the news.

My own contribution was that I had woken up after the operation to be told by the doctor that the operation had been a success, but that there was good and bad news. I asked for the good news first. 'Well,' said the Doc, 'your new heart is in and beating OK.' 'What's the bad news?' I said. 'Well, the bad news is that it was John Wayne's old one!' was the reply. I know it was a bit crummy, but it was the first joke I made about it.

However, in the ward we were all pretty naïve about it and didn't really know the first thing about heart transplants, so I asked John, the charge nurse, about Cambridge: 'Who does the operations?' 'I haven't got a clue,' he said, 'but I have a feeling its a fella called Magdi Yacoub, and that he's as mad as a March hare because he thinks nothing of working through until two in the morning and then going to start his clinic. He's that dedicated a worker.' None of us had heard of Papworth, so I must apologise now to Mr Yacoub for I did not know then that he did *not* operate at Cambridge, and also to Mr English as I didn't know that *he* did!

Later, when John and I were talking, he asked me if I had any worries about going to Cambridge for that sort of thing. Of course, I hadn't. I told him that if they thought I was some sort of guinea pig they would be mistaken! I would soon suss things out and find the back door of the cage. I must emphasise, however, that no thoughts of experimentation entered my mind. I knew this was a genuine attempt to do the best thing for me.

Still, while we had all these discussions about going up to Cambridge, other events were happening in the ward. There was a poor old boy called Trevor who was getting very wound up. They kept on postponing his by-pass operation. It wasn't his first operation by any means, but it was very disconcerting for him to have his date put back all the time. There was another patient who was so disturbed about going down for his operation that the staff began to get a bit worried about it. He had to have a catheter test beforehand and, at the time, St George's couldn't do these tests because of all the alterations, so he was going to have it done at Charing Cross Hospital. However, the doctors soon realised that he couldn't take two visits to the theatre, one for the catheter examination and the other for the operation—it just wasn't on for this particular patient. He is the only patient I know who had his catheter test done in Charing Cross in the morning and then, whilst he was still woozy from the anaesthetic, had his condition checked and then was whipped down to the operating theatre at St George's in the afternoon, to be given a new valve!

As soon as I was told the date of my trip to Papworth, a fellow patient with heart trouble, Tom O'Malley, said to me: 'I know that the day of your journey is your pearl wedding anniversary and you can't get out to get Doreen a present, so I hope you won't be offended by what I'm going to say. You helped me so much over my op that I would like Lou [his wife] to buy a pearl pendant for you to give to Doreen on condition that you don't tell anyone in the ward and you don't give it to Doreen until after I've been discharged.' I happily complied with Tom's wishes as he is such a kind man. To this day, Tom is very happy and is enjoying life and all the nice simple pleasures which go with it—I never cease to wonder how marvellous open heart surgery is.

5

The build-up to the op

The next few days seemed to fly by. The day of my journey to Cambridge arrived. Doreen was going to visit me in the morning, before I left. However, if she didn't make it in time, Maggie was going to give her the full address of the hospital where I was going. She also put a piece of paper in my hand which said 'Papworth Hospital, Papworth Everard, near Cambridge'. It was the first time that I had ever heard of it.

As I was being wheeled out of the ward, Dr Robertson came and put two big blobs of cotton wool in my hands. 'What's that for, Doc?' I queried. 'Oh,' he said, 'they aren't for you. They're for the other doctors at Papworth to stuff in their ears when you start chattering to them!'

Unfortunately, there was a petrol crisis on at the time and petrol was in short supply. Therefore, instead of going to Cambridge in an ambulance, I had to take the ambulance to King's Cross Station, and from there take the train to Cambridge. Nurse Debbie, a very beautiful young girl, came with me, for reasons which I will explain later. We had a cup of coffee on the train going up and when we arrived at Cambridge, for the sake of somewhere warm to sit, we went to the bar. I fancied a drink and so did Debbie. I had a gin and tonic and I think she had a Martini and something. Meantime, Debbie had rung Papworth hospital to get an ambulance to take us up there. The hospital staff were a bit perplexed. They didn't know anything about our travel arrangements and thought St George's had arranged it all. They said they had no ambulance to spare for an hour and a half and instructed us to stay where we were and telephone again then. With my new sense of freedom, I was only too willing to oblige! We had a few more drinks—no harm in that—and Debbie again rang Papworth. It was the same story—stay put and ring again in another hour and a half. I was very happy about this, having newly acquired the taste for gin and tonic, but Debbie said: 'No, Keith—you'd mustn't overdo it.' We passed a very nice few hours there in the station bar and, sure enough, after a further hour or so, our transport duly arrived. In we got for the 12 mile journey to Papworth. It was quite amusing because Debbie had to sit on my

50

lap—on my poor old swollen legs!—as our transport to Papworth turned out to be their kitchen van! The pigs' swill was still in the back of it! What an entrance.

On arrival, I was put straight to bed and then came the problem of the return journey for Debbie. Alma, the Ward Sister, and Beryl Whitehead, the social worker, were both trying to make arrangements for Debbie. Now Debbie was in 'civvies' and they did not realise that she was a staff nurse. They thought she was my daughter, and a rather ungrateful daughter at that, as she was being somewhat unco-operative about their efforts to take her to Huntingdon station, which was the nearest station to Papworth. She was also turning down their offer of a return ticket to London. They were beginning to get a little hot under the collar at Debbie's attitude. Debbie went off to get a cup of tea and, in her absence, I made it clear to the others that Debbie was a nurse from St George's, and the other nurses had juggled their time off to enable Debbie to escort me and then visit her parents, who lived in Cambridge. She therefore didn't want to go to Huntingdon station, she merely wanted to get to Cambridge, meet her mother at five o'clock, spend a few days with her and then buy a single ticket back to London. Debbie's requirements being duly met, I settled down into Papworth Hospital.

Doreen was to travel up the next day—she had to be assessed too—so she was going to stay with our eldest daughter, Jackie, near Northampton. This was 40 miles across country, but more preferable to Doreen than staying in digs or travelling up and down from London all the time.

I suppose the next day was the most important day for us, because it was then that we had to meet Mr Terence English and Dr Petch to 'sell' ourselves to them. All the tests would follow this meeting, although they must have known quite a bit about me clinically by now. I had a chat with both men the following morning, but basically it was Doreen who saw them on her own. During this time, I was sitting on a seat by a lovely pond which was just outside my ward. Soon, I saw Doreen come out of the door. She gave me the thumb's up sign, and was grinning broadly. She seemed to be saying: 'Well, I've done my part, now it's your turn.' Then, when she reached me she said: 'Come on, now they want to see the pair of us.' In we went.

You must appreciate that every patient who goes to Papworth for assessment is trying to grab his only chance of life, so you really do your best to convince the doctors that you should be accepted. I can remember waffling on, saying that I might not be a good clinical bet, but if we were talking in cricketing terms, I would be happy to be fifth wicket down—or something like that. Mr English, I think, has the tendency to speak to you with more caution than he feels. He tells you that the odds are more stacked against you than you think. That's how I see it anyway. I may be totally wrong. Anyway, in the end, Dr Petch

51

had a reservation about my duodenal ulcer. He said he needed a couple of days to evaluate how much the ulcer would conceivably play up, once I had a new heart, with healthy blood pumping round. He told me I would have a decision in three days' time. As we came out of that interview, I asked Doreen how she thought we had done. 'Well,' she answered, 'I think we have done the best that we can.' I told her I thought Mr English was sold all the way down the line, but I was not too sure about Dr Petch. 'Anyway,' I said, 'I have all the time in the world over the next three days to think of counter-arguments.'

To my intense surprise, Dr Petch came to see me a couple of days later and started talking about a heart transplant. 'Look, Dr Petch,' I said, 'what is it going to be—yea, nay or do we lock horns?' He took the wind right out of my sails by saying casually: 'Oh, its yea, of course.' That was it.

So, once more, it was back to clinical tests. During one test, it was found that I had an enlarged and split spleen—no one had been aware of this up to then. It seemed to me that everyone in the place was doing tests on me. They wanted to know my complete medical history, but naturally everything hinged on this duodenal ulcer. Andrew Thorpe, the Surgical Registrar, asked me one day for more details of it. When did I first get it? What hospital dealt with me? etc, etc. They needed to check right back. I told them there was a way of short circuiting this. 'On Monday,' I said, 'there is a doctor joining Addenbrooke's hospital, I believe in Paediatrics, and his name is Bill Brough. Now he is the chap who knows more than anyone about my ulcer. Why don't you wait until he has settled in and ring him up?' Andrew Thorpe grinned, 'I've got a feeling we can short circuit your short circuit!' he laughed, 'because Bill Brough is *not* joining Addenbrooke's, he is in fact joining Papworth Hospital on Monday, as one of your registrars on the surgical team, and what is more, he is visiting the ward tomorrow [Sunday]—so you'll be able to see one of your old chums again!'

Ever since my first visit to Professor Pilkington I'd said to all my doctors: 'Don't worry about me dying, I'll either dance on your grave or do a headstand on your urn according to your method of departure.' I'd told them that I had their name on *my* list. Since I had been treated by him before, Broughie's name had been on my list for quite a while. On the Sunday, Andrew Thorpe introduced him to the others in the ward. Broughie eventually arrived at the bottom of my bed saying: 'Don't tell me—bed 11, St James's hospital, Ward 1—I know!' 'Never mind that,' I laughed, 'Do you realise that you have now buggered up my "Demise List"? I've got you down twice now—which booking do you want, the first one, or this entry which may give you a bit more time?' Broughie laughed and, for a new doctor on his first visit to his new hospital, gave an absolutely unprintable reply! But I was so glad to see Bill and, to be honest, I regarded him as something of a talisman for me. I think that if the occasion arose and I ever had to have another transplant, I would like to think that Broughie was there in attendance. Although I am not all that superstitious, he seemed something of a good luck charm as far as I was concerned. He was most interested to know how I had found out that he was going to Paediatrics at Addenbrooke's. I told him I made it my business to check up on all my doctors, but the truth of the matter is that, just before I left for Papworth Hospital, Barbara had visited me from St James's, had brought me a box of chocolates and had told me all the news, in particular where Broughie was going.

At Papworth, whilst undergoing the tests and routine of the hospital, I also met Harry Lowe, who was also there for a transplant assessment. Now, let me clear up some misconceptions about people who are put forward for assessment. You must understand that, for all these people, it is absolutely their last chance of life. The patient has therefore to be objective, but has to do his utmost to get that important answer 'yes' from the doctors. The question I am most asked about my operation is 'Were you frightened of the operation, once the decision was made?' My answer to this is expected to be: 'No. I had my back against the wall and it was Hobson's Choice. Either the operation or death.' This certainly was *not* true in my case. It was always, for me, a question of having total faith in my doctors. Both Doreen and I had such a positive faith in them that we thought nothing could go wrong. How naïve we were I don't know. It's all water under the bridge now but the relief, then, of getting the decision 'yes' enabled us to really enjoy that first visit to Papworth.

The hospital is set in marvellous grounds with hills and woods all around, and the pond gave us a great deal of pleasure. I remember, when I first saw the hospital, that the rose arbours were just beginning to come into their own. To add to this, in the ward, there was a very interesting collection of patients.

Dr Smailes was one of those patients. He used to get a bit wound up about the fact that the television was always on, although none of us were really watching it, and used to ask continually for us to turn the damned thing off. This we did willingly. I also had to remember not to be too bouncy myself, as I was the only one at that time who had not had an operation—the others were all post-operative patients. Dr Smailes himself had not long returned from the Intensive Care Unit following an operation, and in a further few days he had to go down again for a follow-up operation. So he, in particular, was none too interested in television.

Now, Dr Smailes was an expert on the history of Oliver Cromwell. I am sure he knew more than anyone else about the disappearance and reappearance of Cromwell's head, an age-old mystery to all historians. I remember one night, when Len Sugg, Donald Sproatt and myself, all had quite a conversation about this. This turned in to a real lecture as Dr Smailes was in fact a lecturer. We were so enthralled and spellbound that we didn't realise that time was slipping by, until the nurse came to remind us that it was about 2.30 am and it was time we all got into bed! I have seen Dr Smailes since. He and his wife visited me in the 'bubble', just after my transplant. I saw Donald, too, who was a Bursar at one of the Cambridge colleges. He joined me later on at one of the Papworth fêtes. The only chap I haven't seen since my stay at Papworth is Len, but no doubt, in the future, I shall bump into him somewhere.

I began to notice a behaviour pattern in the post-surgical patients at Papworth, which I hadn't noticed in St George's. Sometime later, when I bumped into Percy in London, I asked him to cast his mind back to Harris Ward and try to remember if the patients, following their operation, often cried. He couldn't remember anything like that happening, whereas at Papworth it was not unusual to see post-operative patients weep. I soon found out that this happened to everybody. I didn't know whether this was due to a slightly different drug used in Papworth to that in St George's or what, but logically it is something to do with the tear ducts. I would say to anybody finding themselves in this position and who are somehow ashamed of the fact— don't worry, it happens to everybody. Its just a natural chemical reaction.

After all my tests had been completed, it was time for me to return to London. The arrangement was that I was to return to Papworth every fourth weekend (between Thursday and Sunday), just for further checks to keep tabs on my clinical condition. However, nobody had actually gone into detail about exactly where I was going. So Doreen and I went home. I must be fair, St George's had told Papworth that they would do everything in their power to co-operate all down the line. I could have stayed in St George's all the time, or just during the week when they would discharge me for a weekend 'pass' at home. But Doreen and I went home, knowing that should anything untoward happen to me, I could go to St George's immediately. It was wonderful for me to get back, in a very limited way, to my local art group and enjoy the activity which was my passion, painting.

Those first days of returning home, following your acceptance for surgery, is the most harrowing time for any patient because you are terrified of missing the boat. Everywhere you go, you have to leave messages of your whereabouts, just in case the hospital needs to contact you very urgently. However, during my period back at home, I did return to Papworth—not as a patient, but to attend the hospital fête. (This was where I again met Harry Lowe and had a little chat in the beer tent with him—more about that later.) Then it was home again.

After a couple of weeks, it was time for my first four-weekly check-up at Papworth. Theoretically, I was due to leave on the Sunday. I was told that Mr English would like to see me, but he was away, and couldn't return by the Sunday. Doreen and I had all the time in the world, so we agreed to stay until the Tuesday. I thought, at that time, that I knew every hospital conspiracy, so I had been really dumb when 'TE' (this is what we called Mr English) said: 'Keith, you know why we have kept you in, don't you?' My face must have been a picture and he continued: 'We didn't tell you that there was a possibility of a transplant this weekend, because we were unsure about the tissue match of the donor heart and we didn't want to build your hopes up. We made up a little cover story to keep you here.' However, this was not to be—my very first disappointment.

Doreen and I returned to London, and a fortnight passed. Suddenly, there was a phone call from Mr English. 'We think we have a possible donor for you,' he said. 'I've had verbal permission from the next of kin, but now I have to go to see them to get the necessary written permission. This will take about an hour and a half. In that time, could you arrange to travel to Papworth, without getting yourself in too much of a state?'

I wasn't sure how to go about fixing these arrangements, so I rang St George's and got hold of Maggie. She said she didn't have a clue as to how to go about getting an ambulance to go to Papworth, but assured me that in an hour and a half's time, if I still wanted transport, she would have an ambulance on my doorstep within ten minutes, or else she would take the afternoon off and drive me there herself. Now, when you consider that for the past seven years Maggie had unsuccessfully been trying to pass her driving test, it would have been a somewhat hilarious drive up to Cambridge! Maggie asked how Doreen had taken the news. I told her that Doreen was over the moon with excitement. Maggie advised me to calm her down and give her a good, stiff sherry (although Doreen doesn't drink) and, she added: 'have one yourself.'

After a couple of hours, the telephone rang and it was Mr Cooper, the Senior Registrar at Papworth. 'It's bad news, I'm afraid,' he said. 'It's all off. The donor's next of kin have changed their minds.' I was repeating these words to Doreen as he was speaking. She looked dumbstruck, and literally collapsed on the couch, unable to understand what was going on around her. Her hopes had been raised so much, and this news was like a bolt out of the blue to her.

The first disappointment, when I was in Papworth, wasn't so bad because we had no build-up of expectation. But this was the disappointment which really knocked the stuffing out of us. This was the one that hurt and really upset us. Anyhow, I suppose it was good training because we were able to treat subsequent 'chances' differently. We would grin to each other and say: 'Oh well, there will be another time.'

When Doreen had got over her shock, we talked about it. We decided that it certainly looked as if Papworth was considering me for an urgent transplant should they find a donor heart with a perfect tissue match. Doreen said: 'I'm not staying down here in London. Let's go up to our Jackie's and stay in Northampton. At least we will be nearer to Papworth then and this will possibly improve your chances.' With that, we packed our bags and notified Papworth that from now on they could contact us at our daughter Jackie's home. Kevin, of course, came with us as, fortunately, he was on holiday from school.

Jackie and her husband, Jimmy, lived on a farm It was not a working farm, but more of a home for them, with about four acres surrounding the house. However, there was enough work to keep them busy. Then, a few weeks later, another bolt out of the blue. Mr English 'phoned. 'We think we have one for you, Keith,' he said, 'can you get into Papworth? Please take your time and don't strain yourself.'

We were not going to let this opportunity slip by, but we realised that we would have to go through Bedford just at the peak of the rush hour traffic. We asked our local bobby if there was any chance of the Bedford police assisting us quickly through the town. Of course, the policeman had to check the story. Unfortunately, when ringing Papworth to make his enquiries, he didn't use my name, Castle, but Jackie's married name, Smith. They, having no Mr Smith on their books, replied in the negative and the policeman therefore did not contact the Bedford police for us. Anyhow, we managed to get through Bedford without all that much bother and eventually arrived at Papworth Hospital. There was Alma (the Ward Sister) waiting to receive us. She explained to Doreen that nothing would happen that night and that the earliest time for the operation would be sometime the following day. She suggested that Doreen return to the farm and wait for any news there. Doreen and Jackie left and I plunged into the usual routine—a shave and cleanse all over before being transferred to the Barrier Room which was a special sterilised room at one end of the Intensive Care Unit. I shall always remember that, as they put me on a stretcher to take me to the bathroom, for the cleansing preparation, one of the patients who I knew quite well, old Dottie Lethbridge, came up to me and said: 'Keith, I wish you wouldn't go through with this—why don't you call it off?' 'Thanks, Dorothy,' I replied, 'you're a big help, I must say!' 'I still wish you'd call it off,' answered Dot. 'Look, Dot,' I said. 'I'm going to go into this thing laughing, and I'm going to come out of it laughing, no matter what you say. Just you wait and see!'

Once in the bathroom, I had to have a bath and scrub myself thoroughly with what they call a Hibiscrub solution. This was to cleanse the body and remove any possible bit of grime or grease, because the next stage was that my body was going to be completely immuno-suppressed. When I had finished bathing and I had let the staff know, my feet literally never touched the floor from then on. I had to step on to a sterile bath mat and dry myself with sterile towels. They lifted me, resplendent in my gown and overshoes, into a pushchair which had been thoroughly scrubbed, and wheeled me to the door of the Barrier Room. They stopped the chair, and I had to step across the threshold, walk across towels to the bed and then get in.

The first tests were to see if I would be allergic to a new drug. The surgeon injected a minute drop of the new drug into my left arm and a minute drop of the old drug into my right arm. Two small blisters formed and he drew a ring around them. The idea was to see if, after a short while, the blisters enlarged at all. Andrew Thorpe explained that, if I showed no allergies, I would be given the new drug, or if I was allergic to one drug, then the other one would be applied. I wasn't allergic to either, so it was to be the new drug. It was called by a very high fallutin' name *Antithymocyte Globulin* (abbreviated to ATG). This is the standard anti-rejection drug.

Andrew then tattooed two dots on my skin—one on my chest and the other underneath my left armpit. These were the points indicating where the electrodes were to be attached when I had ECGs from then on. It was important that the V1 and V6 electrode were in the correct position so that they could have fully accurate readings. I shall always be able to spot a heart transplant patient because, apart from the scar on his chest, these two dots will be clearly visible for the rest of his life.

I was wired up to all the usual monitoring machines. There were thermometers taped to my toes to get peripheral temperatures, things here and things there. Next, Ray Latimer, the Consultant Anaesthetist, came in to start *his* preparations. He inserted various tubes in different parts of my body to enable him to register arterial pressures and my heart rate. Throughout the night I was on regular, quarter-hourly observations, so sleep was intermittent, but it passed quite comfortably and I was looking forward to my op the next day.

Morning came and, as every patient who is labelled 'nil by mouth' can fully understand, this is the time when you are at your hungriest and thirstiest. The day moved on with various people coming in and out doing tests and checks—but there was no sign of my going down to theatre. Gradually, as the day wore on, I was beginning to wonder if it would ever happen. Eventually, somebody came in and told me that it definitely wasn't on for that day. It was getting dark and too late for the helicopter to fly for the donor's heart—it would be far too dangerous. The operation was postponed until the following day.

The next day dawned and a similar sort of caper went on so I was beginning to wonder what was happening. I forget entirely how it was explained to me, or even who did tell me that in fact the operation had had to be called off. I was told that the intended donor wasn't clinically dead and anyway, because of fears of infection in the donor heart, there was no chance of a transplant. I was taken back along the corridor and into a private room again.

It wasn't too much of a disappointment because, as I said before, the first disappointment is the one which sets you back the most, after that, you get used to it. However, I'd like to state here and now, having heard all the criticisms of heart transplantations, or any other transplants for that matter, with the critics going on and on about the morality of it all and questioning how you judge whether a person is dead or not, that that occasion must have been one when the doctors were *very* tempted to throw the switch and get on with their operation. But, complying with the high standards of British medical ethics, the operation was called off, in spite of everybody really wanting it to go on. Unfortunately, shortly afterwards, the intended donor was pronounced clinically dead, but by then it was too late for the heart to be of any use to me.

I spent a few days swanning round my private room and then it was decided that I could go back to the farm. On the day I was due to go out, most of the surgeons, with Mr Hubbard, the Senior Nursing Administrator, came to see me, offering me their sympathy and saying how sorry they were about the situation. I shrugged it off. 'You win some, you lose some,' I told Mr Hubbard, 'there's always another time.'

My only worry at this stage was that they might decide to no longer persevere with me. I therefore made it clear to the doctors that I was prepared to go through 20 chances even if they were aborted. I rather hoped that this would make them think favourably about my case.

So it was back to the farm for a couple of weeks. Some people in the village were going to go on a medieval outing to Coombe Abbey, Coventry. Jackie and Jimmy had had the tickets for some time, but generously asked if Doreen and I would like to go instead. They thought it would do us good. We readily accepted and had a marvellous evening out. We didn't get home until the early hours of the morning but, surprisingly enough, we were up early the following day. We had planned to build some dog kennels. We set about this task during the course of the day and, towards late afternoon, Jackie had to go into Northampton to get some more materials for us. It was then that the telephone call came through. It was Mr English, asking if I could quietly get myself into Papworth for about 9 o'clock that night. I replied that I could get there by 7, but he told me to take my time and that he would see me at 9. He also wished me all the best of luck on this occasion. Just then, Jackie's car pulled up outside. I went to meet her. She saw by the grin on my face that it was good news. 'Yes,' I said,

'Papworth.' She literally jumped for joy. However, we were in trouble, because Jackie's car was a very old banger and could not be expected to make the 40-mile journey to Papworth. Between us we couldn't muster up any transport. Fortunately, a good neighbour of Jackie's, a farmer, offered to drive us to Papworth that evening.

The same routine swung into action. Doreen was told by Alma to go home, have a good night's sleep and ring again in the morning. For me it was—shave, scrub bath and into the Barrier Room which I was quickly to name 'the bubble'.

6

The operation

There was a feeling all round that this time it was going to be for real. There were a few tests which were not required to be repeated as I had undergone them so recently, but I did make sure that my Hibiscrub was carried out thoroughly. Ray Latimer seemed to be attaching more tubes to me than last time and the other two most involved in my preparation were Bill Brough and a nurse called Felicity. There was no tension in the room, as a matter of fact the atmosphere could be described as lighthearted. We chatted and joked throughout the night. I remember expressing surprise at one time when Felicity came into the room with two blocks of salt—they were shaped just like two little space capsules. I wondered what on earth these were for, so I asked her. 'You'll soon find out! Roll over!' she ordered. There was only one place where she could insert them! I joked that she hadn't left room for any vinegar. Then Broughie passed the urine catheter into me—it felt like a four-inch drain pipe! Those two things were the only unpleasant parts of the preparation which I had to go through.

Early in the morning, I had a thorough bed bath and rested quietly until it was time for me to go down to the operating theatre. The date was August 18 1979. (It was a Saturday as all transplant operations were carried out either at the week-end or at night so that no one could accuse Papworth of interfering with the normal hospital work.) Back at the farm everybody was up and hopping with excitement. They had put on the radio and heard an announcement that a transplant operation was going on at Papworth Hospital. This caught Doreen by surprise; she hadn't expected it to be happening at that stage and had almost prepared herself for another disappointment. She rushed to the telephone to ask Alma how I was. 'My dear,' said Alma, 'nothing's happened at this end yet, we haven't even started.' Just as she was going to replace the telephone, she said: 'Hang on, Doreen—they're just wheeling him down to theatre.' So the broadcast was in error, at that stage, the operation hadn't even started!

The ATG (Antithymocyte Globulin) drip which was started at 3 am was finished by now, hence the transfer to theatre. This drug becomes an old friend to a transplant patient, or rather, this was the case in 1979.

I wouldn't know, but it has probably been phased out now in favour of some other drugs. That's how quickly techniques and treatment are moving at Papworth. The dosage given at this stage is designed to kill off most of the white cells in the blood to suppress the body's natural immunity system against foreign cells. For a period after the operation, the dosage is gradually lowered to allow a certain number of white cells back into the system. Other drugs then take over the job of keeping the best possible balance. So the idea is to suppress enough white cells to prevent the body rejecting the transplanted organ but to try to leave enough in to help fight off any bacteria. Then if, at any later stage, a patient should start rejecting, he gets a quick whack of ATG. Usually most of us seem to have a bit of rejection during our stay in hospital, it seems to be par for the course.

Perhaps, before we get into all the clever stuff of the operation, this would be the best time to explain this rejection and white cell point. A good working early warning sign of rejection is to measure the length of the recorded stroke from an ECG examination. A smaller length of stroke than you normally show means that a deeper investigation (a biopsy) is required. Snippets are taken from the suspected heart muscle or graft and, after freezing, are examined under a microscope. If things are normal the white cells will be evenly distributed throughout the blood, but if the patient has started to produce extra white cells and has commenced rejecting, these cells would tend to cluster around a muscle or graft and attack it. Hey presto, it's as easy as that! All these pundits make such a big song and dance about it, but that's it. Now *you* know as much about it as The Boss. Like 'heck' you do, but at least you now have a fair idea!

Now let's go back to the ATG drip. Giving me this resulted in a minor drop in blood pressure, which did not require treatment. At 9.20 I was anaesthetised which caused my blood pressure to fall. This required an infusion of adrenalin, followed soon after by an Isoprenaline drip. These two drugs were given to stimulate the cardiac contraction and heart rate. Working well so far aren't we? As yet, not a scalpel flashed about in anger and already we've been up the creek twice with my blood pressure dropping. But that certainly was said tongue in cheek because Dr Ray Latimer and his team of anaesthetists are more on their toes watching things than probably anyone else connected with the op. Their whole concentration is on balancing and correcting any fluctuations in the body's chemistry or its functions. One minute coagulating the blood to suit a certain stage, the next minute reversing the procedure, and so on. Plasma was next given to maintain a stable haemodynamic state. (That's what I was told; I haven't got a clue what it means! If any reader looks it up and finds out, please let me know!) During this period I was 'towelled' up ready for the start and was breathing on an artificial ventilator. I am also told that arterial and venous blood pressures were monitored by small cannula inserted in the artery and vein of my wrist and neck respectively. My heart rhythm was also measured and my temperature was taken from the roof of my mouth.

Apart from continued observations there was not a lot to do at this stage until the call came through from Mr English (who had gone to collect the donor heart) that all was OK. So the time was filled out by carefully re-checking the equipment, including all the extra items required for heart surgery, such as balloon pumps, by-pass machines and TE's bar of chocolate—the most essential piece of the lot. There's a story amongst those of us who know him that Andrew Thorpe once 'accidentally' pinched the bar and scoffed it. Actually, if that really had happened it would be a sort of rough justice. *We're* not allowed chocolate so why should our doctors? I found that fact out the hard way. Just after the Op, I was in the 'bubble' nibbling away at two enormous bars of chocolate which a neighbour had given me, when in walked Dr Petch, and naturally I offered him a piece. Far from taking a piece he took the lot and confiscated it! So any hard luck stories of sweets and doctors fall on deaf ears as far as I am concerned. But, suddenly, it was all action again. Here is the breakdown of what happened:

11.44 hours. Word received from Mr English that the donor heart had been removed, that there were no problems and he was on his way back.

11.47 hours. An incision was made along the length of my sternum (breast bone). Then, to me, the wonder bit. An oscillating saw is used to cut the sternum. How this saw works I *don't* know. It cuts through bone but stops at tissue or sinew. Some clever bit of 'Hack and Chekker' action! A large retractor is then used to force the two halves of the sternum apart.

12.05 hours. The pericardium covering the heart was carefully opened and all the major vessels prised and cut away from their adjoining tissue, etc.

12.24 hours. The Boss is back.

12.40 hours. To prevent blood clotting, Heparin was given and a large plastic pipe was inserted into the two large veins entering the right side of the heart and a slightly smaller pipe was inserted into the aorta (the main artery from the heart which distributes blood around the body). These pipes were then connected to the heart-lung machine.

12.59 hours. The donor heart was removed from the cooling box and trimmed to size.

13.02 hours. The heart-lung machine now takes over the function of the heart and lungs. From now on the machine is oxygenating and distributing the blood around the body. The timing starts to get very important. Up till then the donor heart had been without blood for

1 hour 58 minutes, also, the chocolate was getting low and the Co-op wasn't open in the village. The body temperature was cooled to 30 degrees centigrade.

13.15 hours. The old heart is removed and the new heart inserted. That is probably how everyone imagines it. For a start not all of the old heart is removed. There are different methods of putting in a new heart—mine was an 'Orthotopic Homotransplant'. That may sound all chi chi and gay—what a lovely piece of one-upmanship it would be when one is introduced at a function to be able to profer a limp wrist and say: 'How do you do, I'm an Orthotopic Homotransplant myself, what are you?'—but the wording only means 'in the same place', as opposed to a piggy back transplant where the new heart could be sited elsewhere. So once again my luck held. I could have gone up to a big six-footer at a party and said: 'How do you do, I'm a piggy back man myself, how about you?' The result would have been disastrous.

However, back to trying to explain the swop part simply. Imagine two 'two-up and two-down' houses, one is a donor house and the other, a recipient house. (I was a builder, remember?) They need to be joined leaving just one 'two-up and two-down' house. It's the two lower rooms that are most important. On the recipient house you cut away the bottom rooms and the front half of the upstairs rooms, leaving the back walls and part of the ceilings and floors. On the donor house you cut away the upper storey back wall and part of the ceiling and floor. Then join one to the other. Call the upstairs rooms the low pressure atriums and the downstairs rooms the high pressure ventricles and there you have it.

Firstly, the pulmonary artery is cut (this takes blood from the heart to the lungs), when the aorta (taking blood to the rest of the body). These are cut as close to the heart as possible. Then the right atrium is cut across the septum to the left atrium, leaving the back of the chambers (the back house walls) and the pulmonary veins (returning blood from the lungs to the heart) intact. Finally the septum is divided, leaving as much tissue as possible.

13.18 hours. The joining of the two hearts was started. I like to use the wording 'joining' as opposed to 'swop'. 'Joining' implies more than the physical side, more a spiritual fusing of gifts unstintingly given, gratefully accepted and skillfully worked upon. For me, nothing can ever surpass that simple act of pure blind faith on everyone's part that it was for something good. Moralists can pronounce on that subject to suit their own convictions, but they cannot taint it one iota.

13.45 hours. All stitching completed, a coolant was circulated around the back of the new heart to keep it from re-warming. Now, mainly all that remained was to join up firstly the pulmonary arteries then those of the aorta.

14.02 hours. A small catheter was placed into the apex of the ventricle to effect decompression and to assist in removing air from the lungs. Fancy one of us waking up at this stage with the 'bends'!

14.06 hours. The clamp was removed from the aorta to allow blood to flow into the coronary arteries again. The heart had been without a supply of blood for 2 hours and 27 minutes. Timing was well on the button and we still had one bit of choccy left. Re-warming the blood was commenced via the heart-lung machine and all remnants of air were removed from all chambers of the heart using a needle and syringe.

14.10 hours. My heart was given an electric shock and it started beating immediately. The few small leaks discovered were repaired and the catheter-come-vent was removed from the ventricle. For the following 25 minutes my heart was supported by the heart-lung machine while it recovered and full body warming was accomplished.

14.35 hours. For the next 5 minutes the blood flow from the heart-lung machine was reduced and the new heart took over completely. 'Look Mum, no wires!' I was doing it all myself again.

14.40 hours. The heart's pumping output was measured and found to be 5 litres per minute. About right for a resting heart. This subsequently rose to 7 litres per minute.

14.45 hours. A weak Isoprenaline infusion was begun. Although the heart action was perfect, this was a precaution in order to keep the heart rate up to compensate for the lack of nervous stimulation. I now had no trigger to make the heart beat, that had been removed. From now on, and for the rest of my life, it will keep pumping away by intrinsic action. Only the first few transplants at Papworth are like this. It is now common practice to insert a pacemaker at the same time, just as a back-up. Not operating, just there to cut in if required.

14.50 hours. All plastic pipes were removed from their respective sites and Protamine was given to reverse the anti-coagulant effect of the Heparin. Two chest drains were inserted to collect any oozing from the chest cavity and two pacemaker wires were inserted and attached to the donor right atrium. These are for back-up, should the heart slow down during the very early stages. Around about six weeks later TE removed them. He retained the very end pieces that had been inside me for bacterial survey and, believe it or not, Doreen took the rest of the wire and had it made up into the decorative inside of a locket.

The chest spreader was then removed and the two halves wired together. The muscles were stitched up, followed by the skin. I was then placed on to a bed which had been swabbed down with disinfectant and made up with sterile linen. Before the operation, as a joke, I'd insisted that Broughie put in the last stitch, saying that he was bound to make such a complete muck up of it that I would then always have something to moan about! Funnily enough, my scar is neat and straight

Right Me before the operation.

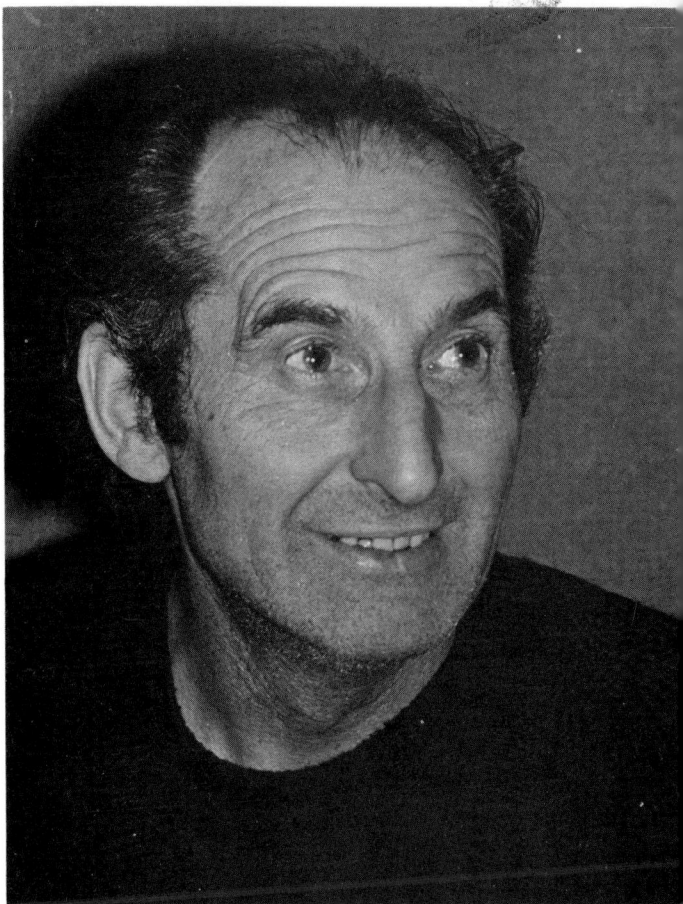

Below I painted this picture of the Barrier Room or 'bubble' with water colours which had to be sterilised first!

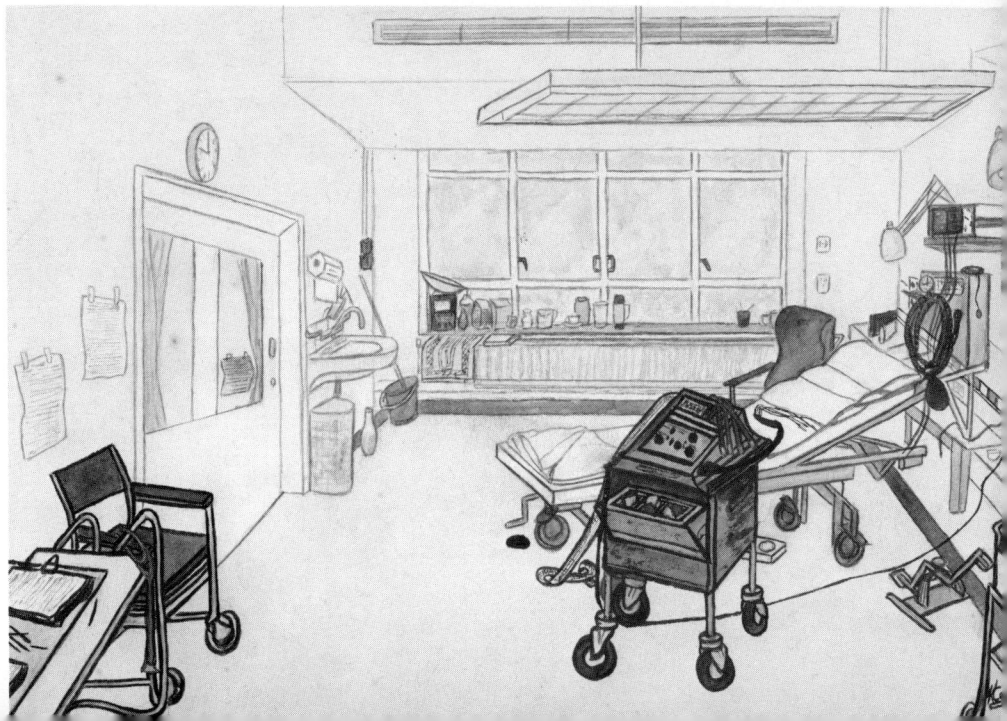

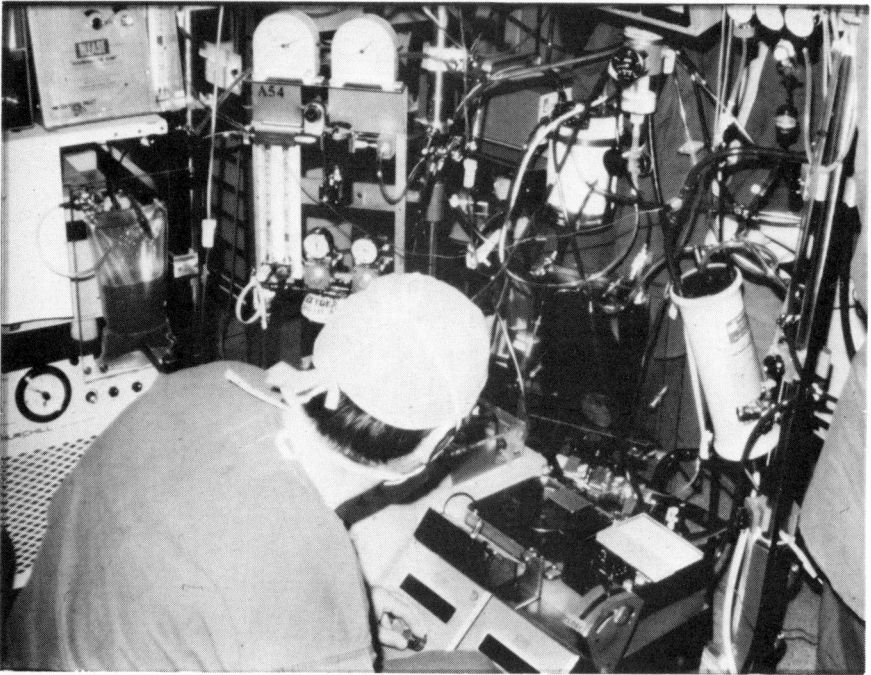

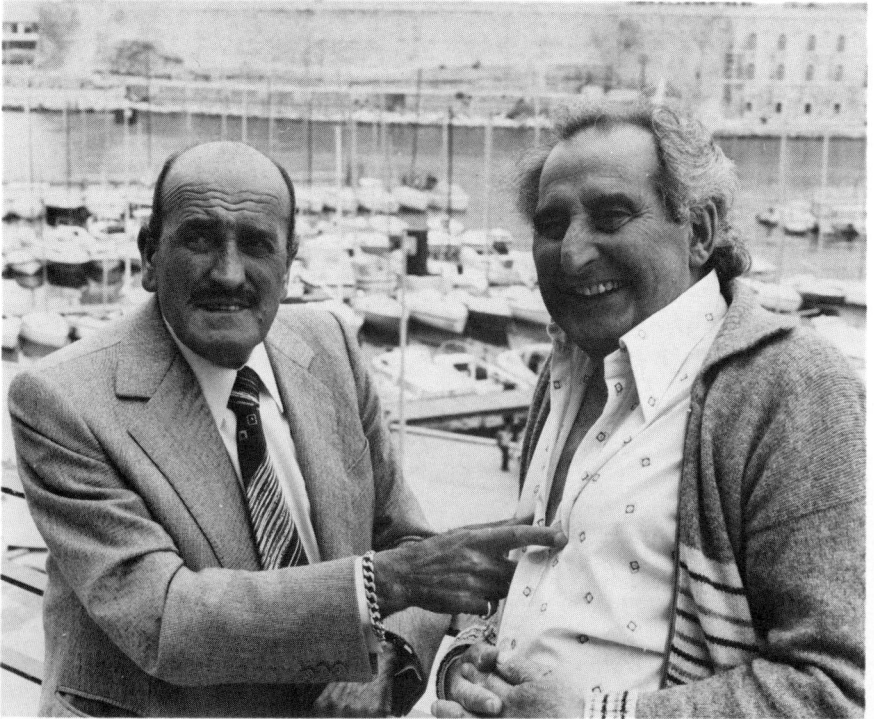

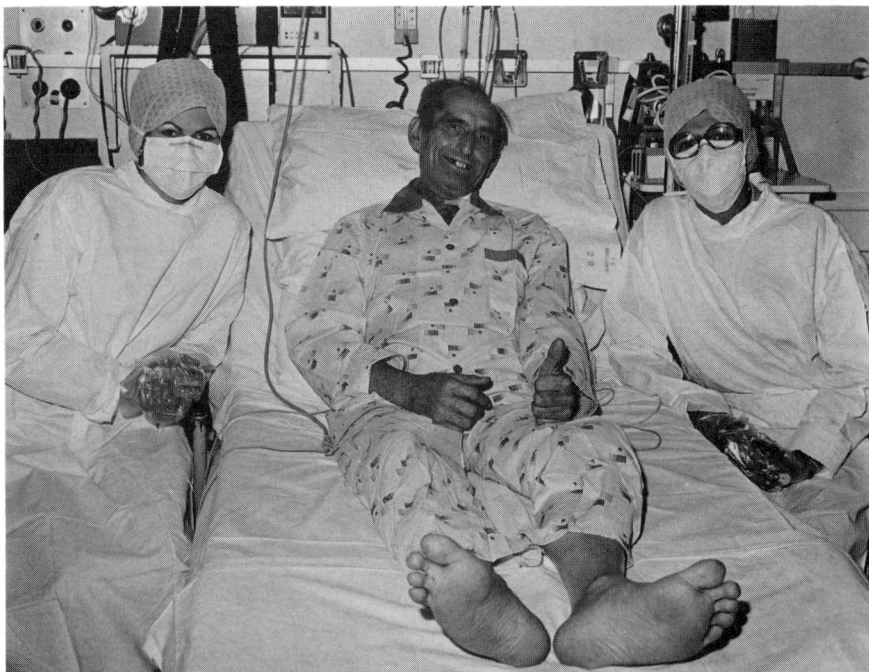

Above left This photograph of the heart-lung machine was taken at the time of my operation *(Papworth Hospital).*

Above This is how Doreen (left) and Jackie had to dress when they visited me in the 'bubble'.

Left Emmanuel Vitrai and me in Marseilles *(Carl Bruin, Syndication International Ltd).*

Right Eddie Kidd jumping over seven heart transplant patients (I'm nearest the camera) at Jock Brand's fête to raise money for Papworth *(Lynn News & Advertiser).*

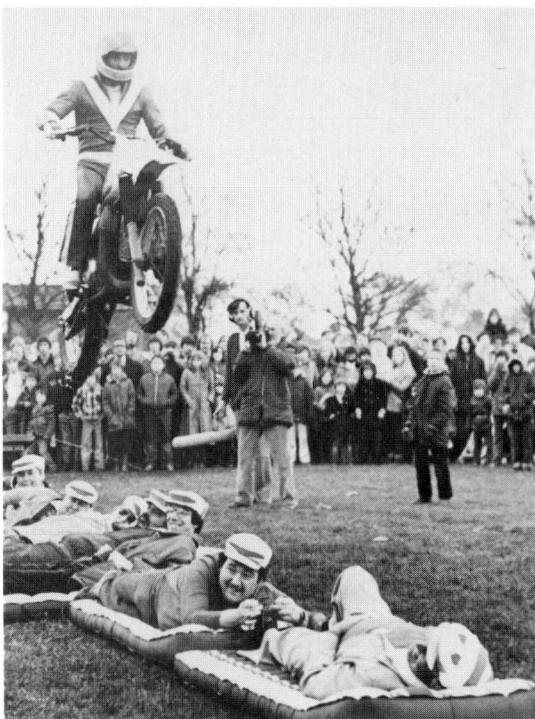

67

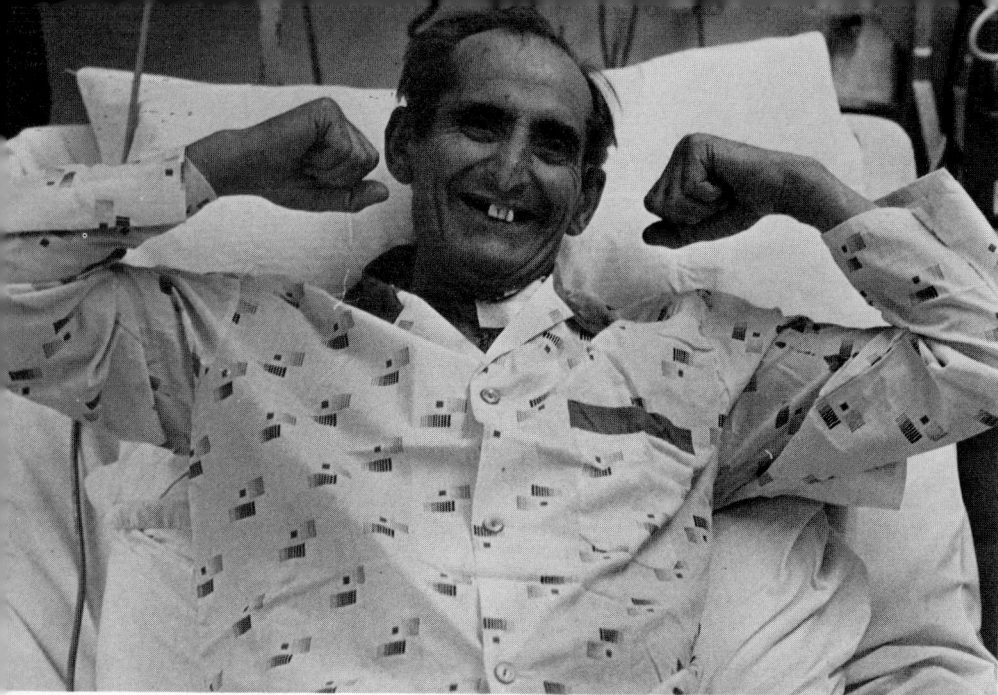

Above It's great to be alive! *(Peterborough Evening Telegraph).*

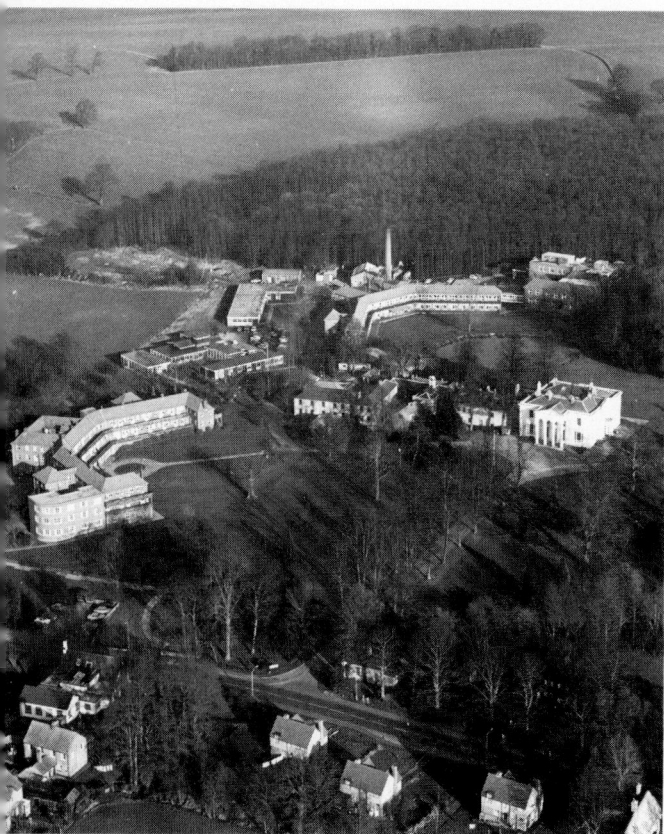

Left Papworth Hospital, Cambridgeshire.

all the way until the last inch when it swings sideways slightly!

Then comes the very last job of the op—looking for the silver wrapping from the chocolate bar. They have never found it yet. I can always tell a heart transplant patient. If they come from Harefield they are as deaf as a post through having to put up with too many of Mr Yacoub's records. If they come from Papworth they all have this mysterious screwed up blob of silver paper showing up on the X-rays. Mind you, Mr Cory-Pearce likes operating whilst listening to *The Old Grey Whistle Test*—apparently he always stomps around. I'm in trouble for that one, he's at Papworth! I won't get away with that Scot free!

So why stick my neck out in the first place? Simple. I've probably been more 'over the top' about my doctors in this chapter than about anyone else because this is the chapter I was a bit scared of writing. I have always tried to avoid being in the position where people could take the opportunity to quote me or use my views as their own. I don't want to get mixed up in medical arguments if I can avoid them. I would sooner leave that to my betters. If anyone is going to use, for their own ends, any quoted facts or figures, in or out of context, this is the chapter they will use. If anyone is silly enough to quote any of the drivel that I've put into this chapter they will virtually be admitting to being as mad as March hares. I have tried to write this chapter about the op as straight as I can, but you must bear in mind that I am as naïve about it as everyone else; I was asleep at the time! Everything I've stated has come from snippets which I have been able to glean since. I just asked Papworth to tell me the approximate times. If anyone tells me that I'm hopelessly wrong about certain facts, they would be correct. I did not keep a diary for future use.

Having justified a very unusual method of writing a chapter it is time to start winding up the op.

17.15 hours. I was wheeled back to the 'bubble' where I was connected to a sterilised artifical ventilator and a new set of monitoring equipment. A nurse was in constant attendance upon me from then on and *all* staff and visitors had to wear sterile caps, gloves, gowns, masks and shoes in my presence. The surgical side was now over with, from then on it was a question of medical treatment—total time from leaving the 'bubble' to returning: 7 hours 55 minutes—a small time in the history of mankind but it meant a bloody great big step forward for me!

7

My second life begins

Naturally, when you come round from an operation you are not lucid and you are very hazy. The first thing that I can remember vaguely is seeing the face of one of the nurses, Avril, floating about around the end of my bed. I think she said: 'Wake up Mr Castle, it's all over,' but I couldn't be too sure. I promptly went back to sleep again. I also seem to remember Mr English bending over me asking how I felt but, once again, I drifted off to sleep. I have it on good authority that, during those bouts of waking up, I was so thirsty that I asked for a glass of milk and was told: 'Later on, later on'. When I again awoke I repeated my request, but still the answer was 'later on'. According to my source of information, I then commented: 'It's a bleedin' long time between later ons!' But I can't remember saying that!

When I was fully awake, I turned to one of the nurses and said: 'What happened? Why didn't the operation go on this time?' She told me that it had taken place. I was amazed and argued with her. She told me to look for myself and, until I actually saw the place, I didn't know I had been operated upon. I had no pain, and what is more, I was breathing clear as a bell. To me that was the most marvellous realisation I have ever had in my life. To be able to breathe freely and easily—I had forgotten what it was like! There is no price which can be put on that feeling. When they asked me to try and cough up a sputum sample, I couldn't cough one up for all the tea in China—my chest was *so* clear and I felt ecstatic about it.

Although I was chattering to people during that day, I obviously still had quite a lot of drugs in me, and I think it took me almost a week to shake off their effects even though I did some physical tests as well during that time. I became more and more lucid as the week wore on.

Naturally, one of my first visitors was John Edwards, the public spokesman for the Heart Transplant team, and from now on he had a really hot potato with me, with the Press continually on his back. I must say a few words about John Edwards. Since my operation and up to the time of writing this book, Papworth Hospital has had more than its share of unfair media coverage, in addition to much praise. It is John who tries to temper this. I think he does a marvellous job. He may have upset some people, when he would not let them go over the top about the op, but he was only doing his job. These people were only looking after their own needs at that time, but John had to look at the overall picture and far into the future to ensure the fairest possible Press coverage regarding heart transplants. He has managed to steer Papworth through some very, very stormy seas and, now that they have reached calmer waters, let's hope that they can get on with their job— which was all they wanted to do in the first place.

A strange remark which I made during my first conversation with John made banner headlines in the papers the following morning. I was feeling so fit and well that I asked him: 'Does anyone know how Fulham got on?' No one knew the score because they had all been too busy the previous night, so John made enquiries for me. Fulham had won 4-3. That made me feel very good. Of course, the papers picked up the fact that my first lucid question following my transplant was about a football match. This wasn't so strange when you consider that for some years beforehand, I would spend my Saturday afternoons, lying in bed, waiting for the football results. I even remember in November 1951, in the Rowley Bristol Hospital, when I woke up after a cartilage operation, I immediately asked how Ivor Broadis had got on, and how many goals had he scored. So you see, my interest in the game was very longstanding, and my questions therefore quite relevant. It is nonsense to assume that, because you have a foreign organ in your body, your personality or interests are going to change—people who think that are talking out of the back of their hat! You don't change the habit of a lifetime and Fulham plays a big part in my life. Many's the time I wish I had remained asleep when I heard the results—but this time it was a good one!

Before I go too far ahead of my story, I must mention that, at the time when I was waking up, I could see some psychedelic lights further down in the Intensive Care Unit. They were flashing mauve and red alternately. I didn't know what they were—they just seemed to weave in and out, with the colours mingling. I was a bit too woozy to register what it was all about really. Subsequently, at various periods, I saw these dancing lights on the ceiling again. I will tell you more about these lights when I get to the place where I eventually found out about them.

During the course of that morning, Doreen, Kevin and Jackie came to visit me. (Keith and my youngest daughter, Wendy, had been caught on the hop regarding the operation and were down in London. Only two of my kids were therefore up with me at Northampton. Keith drove up to be with the family, but Wendy had to stay behind, as she was pregnant.) I first caught sight of them all through the glass sliding door of my 'bubble' or Barrier Room. We waved to each other through the glass and I had a great deal of amusement in watching the antics as they were shown how to get dressed in all the necessary gear in order to come in to see me. Ultra-strict precautions were taken by everyone who entered my room because I was now deprived of all immunity against bacteria. Outside the 'bubble', beside the door, there was a wash basin and also one inside. Anyone entering my room had to wash their hands thoroughly outside the 'bubble', don a protective hat, slip on overshoes (this meant that as soon as an overshoe was on one foot they had to step across the threshold of the room and get the other one on before putting their foot down). As soon as they were inside my room, they had to reach up, take down a surgical gown and put this on as well as medical masks and gloves. It was great fun to watch all this going on!

After the first flurry of greetings, I said something to Doreen which once again hit the headlines in the next day's newspapers. I asked for a Guinness. This is a bit unusual for me, as I don't usually drink it. My visitors didn't stay too long as I was obviously very tired, and there were also a great number of medical checks going on all round me for most of the day. So they adjourned to *Kisby's Hut*, the local pub down in the village, had a ploughman's lunch and came back in the afternoon. Again, I asked Doreen if she had brought me a Guinness. She hadn't thought I was serious, but, back in St George's, Maggie had been giving it to me to build me up, so you see in a way I was asking for it out of habit but how the papers got hold of it I shall never know. Doreen definitely hadn't spoken to a reporter—they didn't even know who she was at that time!

Although throughout this day I could converse with people, I was still very vague about things, although I was aware that the place was becoming like Piccadilly Circus. Although entry to my room was being limited as much as possible, the tests and check-ups on me seemed to be increased every moment. We were now entering the period where, although the operation had been a surgical success, infection and rejection were both very high risks to say nothing of hypertension and shock risks and Mr English was determined that there would be no slip-ups from now on. I was quite woozy although I was aware of certain things, like Jackie saying that Doreen had to go on TV, or at least meet the Press the following morning, and I remember looking forward to seeing my poor old Doreen on the box.

The next day was a Sunday and it passed without my taking too much notice of what was going on. Naturally, I slept a lot, but I did see the psychedelic lights again at the end of the ward, but was not really interested in finding out what they actually were. On Monday it was a busy morning again with all the checks being carried out. An early visitor was John Edwards who asked if I would like to see Doreen on television later on. I naturally wanted to, so he arranged for a television set to be thoroughly cleaned and brought into the room.

John Edwards had been a bit crafty. There was a vast difference between *some* Press which he had asked Doreen to meet, and the great number of people she eventually had to face. Had he been more honest with her, she told me she would never have gone! I think he had also had a word with Jackie because, on the morning they were due to arrive at Papworth, Jackie made a special point of doing Doreen's hair nicely and lending Doreen one of her own outfits. As it was, Doreen looked very smart indeed.

The family arrived at Papworth in a battered old Land-Rover. John nearly had a fit. 'Good gracious!' he exclaimed. 'You can't arrive at the Nurses' Home to meet the Press in that old thing.' So he arranged for a better looking car to take them up there! Doreen nearly had a heart attack when she saw the waiting crowds of reporters and cameramen. They were all over the grass and were swarming around like bees. She almost turned and ran. However, there was one familiar face in that huge crowd. This was a freelance journalist called George who is a friend of our son-in-law, Jimmy. Naturally, he knew, before the other journalists did, the identity of the heart transplant patient at Papworth, but he very fairly did not release any information until the Press had been officially called to meet Doreen. He told us he had struggled with his conscience because he knew he had a scoop, but he was also aware of his allegiance to Jimmy. The nearest he came, was to ask Jimmy down to the local pub to see if, under the influence of drink, he would agree to his leaking the story. Unfortunately for George, Jimmy, although not a drinking man by any means, managed to drink George under the table. George therefore didn't get Jimmy's agreement, and he kept his word. Anyway, good old George sat beside Doreen and made her feel more at home.

Up to that time, the Press had certainly been misled about who the transplant patient really was. One assumes that they had their own way of finding out, but the majority of them, when the story first broke, were well on their way to the West Country under the assumption that it was Harry Lowe. The family had received hilarious reports that, down in London where we lived, the journalists were busy trying to dig up information about me and obtain photographs. I suppose first prize for enterprise must go to the journalist who had heard from another reporter that the transplant patient was an artist from south-west London, put two and two together and went round to the local Battersea Arts Centre, a place I used to visit quite a lot. He conned the receptionist into revealing my first name by saying he was doing a story on me, but she said she couldn't give him any information about Keith, but told him to try my art teacher. She gave him Carol's telephone number. He rang her and said: 'We're doing a story on Keith um . . .

um . . .' 'Castle', said Carol, and then he had my full name!

Another paper gained information in what I consider to be a very sordid way and it wasn't the paper's doing this time. My nephew is a television repair man and was working in someone's house when the news of my transplant was on. He told the person that it was his uncle and how pleased the family were. When he had completed the job, the customer asked him for his name and address, so they could recommend him for further work. As soon as he had left the house, the customer rang a national newspaper and sold the information. He obviously guessed that he had a 'hot' story. I thought that was despicable when I heard about it, but at the time I was oblivious of it all, being nicely cocooned in my 'bubble'.

When Doreen came to see me soon after, she told me she was beginning to get offers from the media for my story. Indeed, not only Doreen had these offers, but the family down in London as well. This was a complete shock to me, because I had never envisaged anything like that. When she told me the amounts they had offered, I went raving mad. Sums of £30,000 were offered. Papers were offering £10,000 more than their rivals. It was unbelievable to me, there I was, only a few short hours after having received a new heart, and being bandied about like a chunk of commercial meat. However, I should state that all the papers were quite nice about it and there was nothing ghoulish in their attitude—it was just to be a happy story and they were very good and kind to Doreen when they had any dealings with her. The Press have always been good to us ever since. But, sadly, we found out later on, that Mr and Mrs Prestt (my donor's parents) during their moment of sorrow, had received the worst end of it and had been hounded mercilessly by the Press. It must have been a very distressing episode for them.

There were occasional laughs when the younger, more adventurous members of the Press tried to infiltrate the hospital and get into my room—but there was no chance of that whatsoever. Each and every devious means was discovered. Doreen and I had a chat in my 'bubble' about the offers. 'No way is any story about this going to be sold like that,' I said. Poor John Edwards was also very worried. He was very concerned that we would make commercial whoopee out of it. Mr English was concerned, too, as these added pressures on me would not do much to aid my recuperation.

By now, I was eating full meals, if that can be the description of what they were shovelling down my throat! No one was quite sure about what sort of diet I should be on and, until that had been sorted out, I was mainly having tinned fruit, and big blobs (about 2 foot thick) of scrambled egg. Naturally, after a few days, I found this food very boring. I asked if they could perhaps liven the egg up by putting a bit of

74

sauce in the mixture. They consulted and agreed.

We had to establish a routine because there was no precedence in Papworth as far as passing things into the Barrier Room was concerned. Food had to be autoclaved which entailed being baked in a tin within a tin at a very high temperature to kill all germs. The nurse concerned would bring the meal up in the outer tin, as far as the sliding door of the Barrier Room. She had to take the lid off and just reach in with her hand and the nurse on duty or I (when I was more mobile) would take the inner tin from the outer tin into the room. All cutlery and crockery arrived in the room wrapped in two layers of sterile paper. The nurses in the outer room would tear off one layer. It was then the practice to throw them the 4 feet or so on to my bed, where I would tear off the inner paper. Everything that had to come into my room was treated in this manner—from drugs to linen.

Naturally, the most important routines were the strict check-ups and observations and doctors' conferences which were going on at the time. Then followed one of those amusing little incidents which shows you that Papworth is such a unique and friendly hospital and which gave me my first fillip about the place. All the surgeons were standing outside the 'bubble', when TE suddenly pointed towards the other end of the Intensive Care Unit. As everyone else turned to look down the ward, TE turned to me and, through the glass, put up his two thumbs as if to say, 'you're doing marvellously.' The funny thing was that, during this little meeting of all my doctors, every time that one of them thought the others were not looking, he gave me a thumbs up sign. Each and every one of them actually did that, and to this day each of them thinks that he was the only one who did it!

TE gave me another morale booster a few days later. He was in my 'bubble' and glanced at one of my monitors. He grinned widely and said to the nurse: 'When did *that* appear on the screen?' He was obviously pleased with whatever it was. The nurse replied that it had been showing for some time now, and she assumed that he had known about it. I still don't know the significance of the conversation, but I did know that if it was a good sign for TE then it was a good sign for me, and it made me feel very good indeed.

It was then—36 to 48 hours after the operation—that I had my first little setback. I suddenly had diuretic problems and was unable to pass urine. My liver had always been a cause of worry and, before the operation, it had literally ceased to function—actually it would probably have been my liver which would have caused my death in the long run, because it was so bloated and distended. Mr English consulted with the Renal Unit and, amongst other remedies, it was suggested that my fluid intake be reduced. It was not so drastic as it had been back in St George's, but it was considerably reduced. After a few days the problem righted itself, and I wasn't troubled again by this.

Two things then happened simultaneously. I noticed a new phenomenon in the room and I found out what the flashing lights were, down at the other end of the Unit. The first thing was the clock in my room. It was above the door opposite my bed, high up, and slightly to one side of my line of vision. It had a round face and, apart from being five minutes slow, which annoyed me intensely, the second hand was brilliant red. When this hand swept round the convex surface of the clock, optically it seemed to bend backwards like a bow, and when it passed the concave surface it would seem to spring back. This was repeated over and over again, naturally. On the following Wednesday, I did in fact, when no one was looking, get up on a chair, take the clock off the wall in order to wind it on five minutes. The rawlplug holding the hook for the clock was loose, and I was busy fumbling, trying to get the blessed clock back on the wall without being seen. Unfortunately, one of the surgeons came into my room and saw me. He gave me such a telling off and threatened me with punishment from Mr English. I was frightened to death—but I don't think he ever told him! What he didn't realise was that I didn't consider my action as foolhardy as he obviously did. You see, all my life I had been a builder and was well used to heights, and to me simply standing on a chair was the same as being on solid ground. However, I realise that even falling 2 feet could have been extremely dangerous for me at that time and I suppose I shouldn't have done it.

Now I was to find out what those flickering lights were. It turned out to be my only criticism of Papworth Hospital. Papworth is a marvellous place and I have a great deal to thank them for, but I do make this criticism. It appeared that some sort of light fitting was hanging over Sister's desk. In actual fact it turned out to be segments of white fire clay bars, similar to gas fire bars. 50 per cent of the bars would glow with an ultra-violet light in order to trap all the various insects flying around. The bees, dragon flies and other flies would be attracted to the ultra-violet and fly close to it. Soon after, the ultra-violet light went off and the rest of the bars would give out an intense infra-red light, which literally singed the things to death. It was the most hideous thing that a patient recovering from an operation could possibly sit and watch. Whoever invented the device I don't know, but it must surely have been a consortium comprising Roland Emmet and Dracula using the plans drawn up by Ronald Searle. I spoke to Dee, one of the staff, about it and she said it was a new fangled thing which had not been installed for very long. The staff found it a bit much, too, so I don't think it was used much after that. They didn't like having roasted insects falling on their heads every few minutes. Snap, crackle and pop for breakfast may be commonplace, but that was ridiculous!

The most hilarious thing happened to me shortly afterwards. I think it was the funniest experience I had during the whole time I was in the 'bubble'. It was far funnier than any situation comedy on the television, and surely it could only happen in Britain, and in particular, to the British National Health Service. It happened like this. One day there was a great flurry of activity outside my 'bubble' and the lab technician came bounding in. In his intense excitement, he had forgotten completely to scrub up and don his protective clothing. 'Keith,' he asked, 'have you been taking that powdered egg with the sauce in it that you asked for a few days ago?' 'Yes. Why?' I answered. 'For God's sake don't eat any more,' he advised, 'also, don't talk about this incident when you get out, or the makers of the sauce concerned will have to sue you in self defence.' He went on to explain that he could grow better cultures on that particular sauce than from any bacteria which was on the floor. He couldn't do it with any other make of sauce, so that one must have some ingredient in it that the others didn't. So, I won't divulge the name of this particular sauce but, if all the sauce manufacturers in the country would like to write to me to prevent me from naming their product one day, I will oblige, provided they make a donation to Papworth Hospital! It was also a spin off from a heart transplant that the hospital has now got a cheap method of growing cultures—all they have to do is tip 'Brand X' sauce on the floor!

By now, I was in the middle of all the medical changes which were going on within my body, as the result, I assume, of having fresh healthy blood pumping round me. One of the things was that I was able to write letters again. However, this was not without great difficulty—because I gripped the pen so tightly it stiffened my wrist and I was unable to make natural curve movements. I therefore had to use my whole arm. I assumed it was the strength coming back into my fingers and the fact that I had not yet been able to adjust my hand for normal writing.

Another thing was that all the noises in my head became over-exaggerated. The most marvellous one of the lot was when they were taking my blood pressure. As the nurses used to let the mercury fall in the gauge, after pumping it up, it was just like a firework exploding in my head. These noises lasted about two weeks before tailing off completely. However, I had been used to a continuous headache after my first heart attack. This headache lasted for nine months then disappeared, leaving a continual singing in my ears, right up to the time of the operation, so these other noises made a pleasant change! I still get singing noises to this day, but I don't worry about it.

Then there were the cup handles! Once again, with the strength returning to my fingers, I seemed to be snapping the handles off the cups as soon as I picked them up. I was like Superman, but it was a terrible nuisance for the nurses. All these little odd things went after about two weeks, but I just couldn't get over my fingertips. I used to hold my hands out to Jackie and say: 'Just look at my little pink cherries!' You see, up until that time, my hands were blue and lifeless-looking but after the op they turned a beautiful pink. I have never got over that little miracle to this day.

On about day three after my operation, Fulham were on the box playing football. Naturally, I settled down early to watch that match. Now, I don't know whether or not my surgeons will disagree with me as I have never discussed this point with them, but I think it was because I still had so much of the drugs in my body that the game appeared to be much more detailed and almost seemed like a slow motion affair to me. The highlight of this was, during the course of the match, that the opposition got a penalty award. Pop Robson took the penalty, and he's no mean slouch at doing those sort of things, and the goalkeeper didn't even smell the ball as it slammed into the goal. However, as far as things appeared to me, from the moment that ball left his foot it was just dolly-lopping along the ground, and if I had been the goalie I would have had time to fry half a dozen eggs, eat them, and still had ample time to put my hand out and stop the ball!

By now, Doreen could make arrangements for Kevin to attend the local school in Northampton, as it was obvious that the family would be spending some time in the area. Jackie and Doreen settled into a some-what arduous routine. They would get up first thing in the morning and see to the animals, make breakfast for Kevin and for Jackie's daughter, Samantha, and pack them off to school. After a bit of housework it was into the car for the 40-mile journey across country to Papworth to see me. They used to arrive about lunchtime and spend as long as they could with me in the 'bubble', before they had to leave for the journey back to Northampton in time to collect the kids from school.

Obviously, in those early cautious days of my recovery, I was left alone in the 'bubble' whilst I was eating a meal. Unfortunately, this coincided with the only possible time that Jackie and Doreen could visit me and, at first, the nurses used to try and make them wait outside. There was one occasion when they had to wait outside for about an hour and a half, they then had only about a quarter of an hour's visit before they had to make that long return journey. Doreen was a wee bit upset about it and told me. I had a quiet word with the nurses and explained the situation. The nurses were very understanding and after that they allowed Doreen and Jackie in, even when I was eating.

Food became a bit of a thing with me after that. I had never been a big eater. Sid, the chef, knew the type of menus which I was allowed to have, and did his best to please. When the meals arrived they were the most gargantuan meals that anybody could wish for, far too much for me. The nurses were rushed off their feet most of the time and I tried not to be a bother to them. When it was time for my breakfast, I would say: 'Don't worry—just give me a cup of tea and I'll have my breakfast when you're less busy.' So, on a couple of occasions I had my breakfast at 10 o'clock and then at 12 o'clock I was given another huge meal for lunch. This was followed by another huge meal at 5 in the afternoon, with nothing else until breakfast the next morning. To me it was a bit stupid because I felt as if I was being force-fed. Mr English wanted me to eat good meals to keep my strength up but my stomach couldn't cope with such large amounts.

I was on restricted fluids of 2,000 cc a day, so Doreen brought in a flask and the nurses measured the amount of tea it contained. So, the girls didn't ever have to worry if they were very busy, as they knew I had a cup of tea handy. Then, when the rush was over, I would give them the flask so they could measure what amount I had taken from it. This became our routine and I preferred this system because it meant that I could choose when I had my liquid intake throughout the day.

The only other thing I missed in the ward was a mirror. It was an unfortunate oversight and too late by that time to get one put up on the wall, so for the next eight weeks I had to use a small handbag mirror, sellotaped on to the window, but it wasn't very big for shaving purposes, I must admit!

From this time, half way through the first week, to the end of the week, events were to take on a more hilarious turn. Doreen had now become used to visiting me in the 'bubble' and was more accustomed to the rather strange surroundings and, thinking she was helping me by keeping things sterile, she would go round swatting all the wasps and insects that flew into the room. The fact that they shouldn't have been in at all was another story—but they always managed to get in somehow. I used to tell her to stop amusing herself by swatting all these dead bodies on to my nice sterile floor, but she never did see what she was doing!

My next moment of enjoyment came with the Viennese night of the Promenade Concerts. I was determined to lie back lazily and enjoy the concert. I got rid of the nurses, who had put out the commode for me, drew the curtains and sat on that commode for the complete duration of the programme! I don't know how many other concert goers make a regular habit of sitting on a commode, with their trousers around their ankles, listening to their favourite pieces of music, but for me it was a marvellous one-off experience! I couldn't help but think that, if Sir Malcolm Sargent conducted the programme with his trousers around his ankles, he would certainly be living up to his nickname of 'Flash Harry'!

Doreen used to leave some money for me on the nurses' desk because I was literally unable to touch it at that stage. It was definitely, for me, filthy lucre! One night, Dee and the rest of the night staff had arranged to have a Chinese takeaway from St Neots. They invited me to participate. They asked Mr English if this was all right and he made it conditional on the Pathology Lab agreeing, as they did. I have no doubt that my particular portion was autoclaved. So there I was, in the early hours of the morning, inside my 'bubble', enjoying my Chinese meal and a couple of glasses of vino which went with it, reading a paper which reported Mr English's cautious reports that if I was alive in three months' time, I would stand a fair chance of leading a normal life!

On another occasion, I said to Penny, another nurse, that I felt sure I could smell burning in the room. Now the room was full of all kinds of electrical equipment, so Penny went round, sniffing each and every one of them. She couldn't smell burning so she told Sister. An engineer arrived and, after taking the usual precautions of entry, he checked the equipment too, but couldn't find anything wrong. But he agreed with me, there was a smell of something burning. He decided to go out and start checking all the trunking systems, as there had to be something wrong somewhere. He came back in about two hours, roaring with laughter. 'You're not going to believe this,' he said, 'the ward kitchen discharges into your room, and your room discharges into the Intensive Care Unit. So, though I was supposedly in the Barrier Room, I still had the overflow from the kitchen!

Then came the Friday evening which I shall not forget in a hurry. Penny had just come on duty, slid the Barrier Room door open a few inches and asked if there was anything that I needed for the evening. 'No, thanks,' I answered, 'but I think you had better go and report to Sister that I have done in my cartilage.' There was I, lying on the bed with my knee bent up, unable to straighten it. Penny ran and told Dee, who looked up and immediately started laughing. She sent for the Duty Registrar Surgeon, who happened to be Woggie.

Woggie was a marvellous person. His real name is Dr Wardeken. When he first joined Papworth, the nurses were muddling him up with a character who appeared on television at the time, a Mr Warleggen. Woggie settled things by asking everyone to call him 'Woggie' and I have always called him that. Anyhow, Woggie said there wasn't much doubt that I had cartilage problems. He told me not to worry about it, the most important thing was that I should get a good sleep. He asked me to take a sleeping tablet that night, as he knew I never took anything of that sort. I reluctantly agreed and he said they would get an orthopaedic chap over from Addenbrooke's the next day to look at me. He said they might be able to do something by merely injecting the knee, but that would be up to the orthopaedic man to decide.

The following day, this chap duly arrived with Bob, the Senior Theatre Technician. He looked at my leg and, as Woggie had predicted, he injected the knee, and the leg straightened of its own accord. A true anti-climax. Who would have believed that, within a week of having a heart transplant, I could do in my cartilage? Mind you, I had suffered with this for the past 30 years, so possibly it was just the result of good blood getting to the nerve ends of that particular knee that aggravated the old trouble.

That little episode concluded the first wonderful week of having a new heart. My brain now clear, I was able to sit back and study some of the doctors' idiosyncracies as I was now living in such close proximity to them. Quite naturally, all the doctors involved in my operation, were highly delighted with the results. The two that stuck in my mind were Andrew Thorpe—whose head was so high in the clouds he could have walked into a 10-foot high brick wall, and the other was a young student. He was in such a state of euphoria that he didn't know what day of the week it was! Woggie, as usual, would put himself out to keep me up to date with the latest information about my condition. Mr Cooper, the Senior Registrar, was concerned for me when he saw me mopping up the floor of my room one day. (By this time I was allowed to wash at the sink in the room. Naturally, if I splashed some water on the floor whilst washing, my first reaction would be to get hold of a mop.) I managed to convince him that I was trying to act normally. Eventually he accepted my reasoning. Later, I graduated to mopping my whole room, and secretly, I felt he was pleased that I was keen to get on and do things for myself.

As it was a Barrier Room, the nurses had a tremendous amount of cleaning to do. Windows, walls and surfaces were continually washed, to say nothing of the floor, so it was nice to be able to help the nurses when I was able, by starting with the floors, and eventually within a short period, doing it all myself. It gave me a great sense of achievement.

Now Mr English. He had certain hang ups too! In my room there were some curtains near the sink and people used to take off their protective gowns, put them on coat hangers and then hang them up on the curtain rail. Unless these gowns were pressed tightly against the window, they used to hang right in front of the sink. I soon noticed that Mr English took rather a dim view of this. Consequently, I used to warn the nurses to this effect. TE always had the hump if he saw the gowns near the sink, but in his courteous way he tried to explain to the girls that he wanted these gowns pushed back tidily against the window. One nurse took notice of my warning and saw to it that everything was in order. TE would come in, immediately look to see how the gowns were placed and purr like a kitten if they were in the correct position. Meanwhile, I'd be pulling faces at the nurse and laughing behind his back and calling her teacher's pet! Bloomin' good job he never twigged what I was doing!

In actual fact, there was good reasoning behind TE's obsession with the gowns being near the sink. All sinks have a waste trap and he was, of course, worried that germs would somehow get on to the gowns. Actually, the waste trap was not like ordinary traps. It was covered in copper and, periodically, electric connections to the waste pipe, together with chemicals, would literally boil the contents of the S-bend. That's how thorough they were in their attempt to keep germs out of the room. I must say, although I have been joking about smells and insects getting into the room, I know it is impossible to keep these out, and the staff certainly did their utmost to see that I was in a germ-free atmosphere to aid my recovery.

On the nursing side, it was poor Felicity who had the job of sitting down to listen to my ramblings when I was in the very chatty stage. I had gone through a period of hiccupping which caused laughter all round, but my chatty stage must have been a real bore for Felicity. I used to sit in a chair, half woozy, chattering on about everything under the sun. I remember one occasion, suddenly coming to and remembering that I was talking about snakes. Felicity must have thought that I was going round the bend, but in fact I was thinking of events in the past and, in particular, a friend of mine from the Navy days. I will digress for the time being from things medical, and tell you this little story which was then in my mind.

I expect that old mate of mine has been telling this story to disbelievers for many years, so, if he does read this book, he will at last have confirmation of its truth! The chap concerned is Geordie Lockhart, from Newcastle. At the time in question, we were in the Far East and a crowd of us from HMS *Vengeance*, the aircraft carrier, had been sent to a rest camp in the hills of Ceylon at a place called Dyatelawa. It was cool up there which helped us to get rid of the prickly heat which had bothered us for a good while. One day, we hired bicycles in the village and decided to have a day out.

We were riding down the steep hill in the village, in single file, when, to our horror, there suddenly appeared the biggest snake I had ever seen. It was so long that it reached across the road from one side to the other—even though the road was a narrow one. I was immediately behind Geordie Lockhart, who swerved, slamming on his brakes to avoid the creature. This didn't work and his front wheel ran over the snake. It wriggled so much that poor Geordie and the bike ended up in the ditch at the side of the road. Meanwhile, I was frantically braking too and, luckily for me, the snake wriggled off into someone's garden, with two natives running after it. However, I also couldn't keep my balance and landed piled up on top of poor old Geordie. A few minutes later, the two natives, who had chased the snake into the garden with no weapons at all, reappeared with it casually slung across their shoulders. It was huge! They wanted to show it off to Geordie and me but we were too terrified even to inspect it. I bet when Geordie tells his friends in Newcastle that he ran over a massive snake on his bicycle he is never believed. I'm here to tell them it really did happen!

Poor old Felicity had to sit and listen to all this and similar ramblings and, one day when Doreen asked her how I was, she replied: 'Oh, he's talking the hind legs off a donkey.' But luckily I soon passed that stage in my recovery.

The other nurse who suffered at my hands was poor old Penny. The Intensive Care nurses were then doing my ECGs. This work was far more involved than the normal ECG examination. After the normal run of the print out there was a great business of undoing certain wires and attaching them to others, and generally it was quite a mathematical problem and poor old Penny used to get hopelessly beaten. I soon twigged what was supposed to happen so, between us, Penny and I usually managed to get a correct read out, but I shudder to think how much wasted paper the National Health Service had to pay for!

I don't know exactly when it was I had my first biopsy, but that was the next big highlight. I was going to have to make the journey between the 'bubble' and the X-ray room which was on a different floor. Every single precaution was taken—it must have been the cleanest route for any man to make. Long before I had to leave the 'bubble', the cleaners scrubbed every corridor and even the lift on my route to the X-ray room. Meanwhile, I had to thoroughly cleanse myself and then the nurses dressed me for the journey. They raked the bottom of the barrel for every bit of sterile clothing they could find. I had on two surgical hats, and how many gowns and sterile sheets there were I don't know, but there seemed to be more and more and more put on me. I had long socks right up my legs and wasn't allowed to stand on the floor, but had again to stand on a sterile towel. With all the gear on I was about 5-foot wide and the nurses fell about laughing at me. The only visible part of me were two little beady eyes peering out from a slit between the sheets. One of the nurses ran to get a camera to record this, but couldn't find one anywhere.

When the time for the 'off' came, they flung open the doors of the 'bubble' and charged with me down the corridor and into the lift. There was a guard on every corner and intersection of the corridor to stop people coming near me and, visitors who were held back were amazed to see this fat little figure being propelled, like a lunatic, down the corridors at top speed.

If Doreen had a shock at the number of people at her first Press interview, then I had a similar one on this occasion. I assumed that I was going to undergo a similar sort of investigation to that one I had had in St George's—just Dr Petch and a couple of technicians and that would be it. However, when I arrived, I had the feeling that all medical personnel from the Cambridge area were present. They weren't just part of the routine team, but had just come to look. The place was flooded with people. Come to think of it, I may have been wrong in my assumption that they were mainly people who had come to watch, they may well have been on stand-by in case of an emergency, as this was the first biopsy of its kind carried out at Papworth. Unfortunately, the patient before me had never reached the stage of being able to have a biopsy. That was poor Charlie McHugh.

Dr Petch commenced the biopsy in his usual calm and unflappable manner. I can distinctly remember the repartee between Dr Petch and Andrew Thorpe to the effect that Andrew was now TE's representative on this planet, as TE had now been elevated to be amongst the gods!

To the uninitiated, this type of biopsy entails a piece of plastic tubing being placed in the jugular vein and a thing called a bioptone being pushed through it to the heart. They take snippets of the heart and the heart muscles for subsequent tests to see if there is any sign of rejection. In this way they can positively see if the body is rejecting the new tissue. There are tests which give you guidelines, but the biopsy is the total proof, and biopsies are a regular occurrence to patients, especially in the early stages. Naturally, Dr Petch was feeling his way, as everybody was. There was just a tiny area of skin around my jugular vein exposed, the rest of me was covered right up, and the big X-ray machine was close to my chest. Underneath the covering gowns, Felicity on one side, and the Theatre Sister on the other, gave me their index fingers to hold on to and I was told to give their fingers a squeeze if anything hurt me. This was because Dr Petch, whilst inserting the bioptone, had to be careful not to take a wrong turning. If he did, the bioptone would touch some part of my vein walls and give me a jolt. In subsequent biopsy examinations, I saw, on 'TV' screens which wree strategically placed round the room, the bioptone actually going down and sometimes they did bump against the walls of the vein. You could actually see Dr Petch curl the wires in order to make a turn down a vein. If I saw on the screen that he had missed, I saw it a split second before I actually felt it and so was forewarned. Biopsy examinations became routine, although, on the first one, when I was not sure of the procedure, I did feel a few little aches and pains inside me. However, with the constant chatter going on, it was nothing really, and I was soon back in the ward. Within 5 minutes I was sitting up eating my dinner.

On subsequent biopsies, Dr Petch began to use easier and easier routes all the time. He used to look at X-rays of the complete arterial system of my body (to my mind, it was rather like looking at a map of

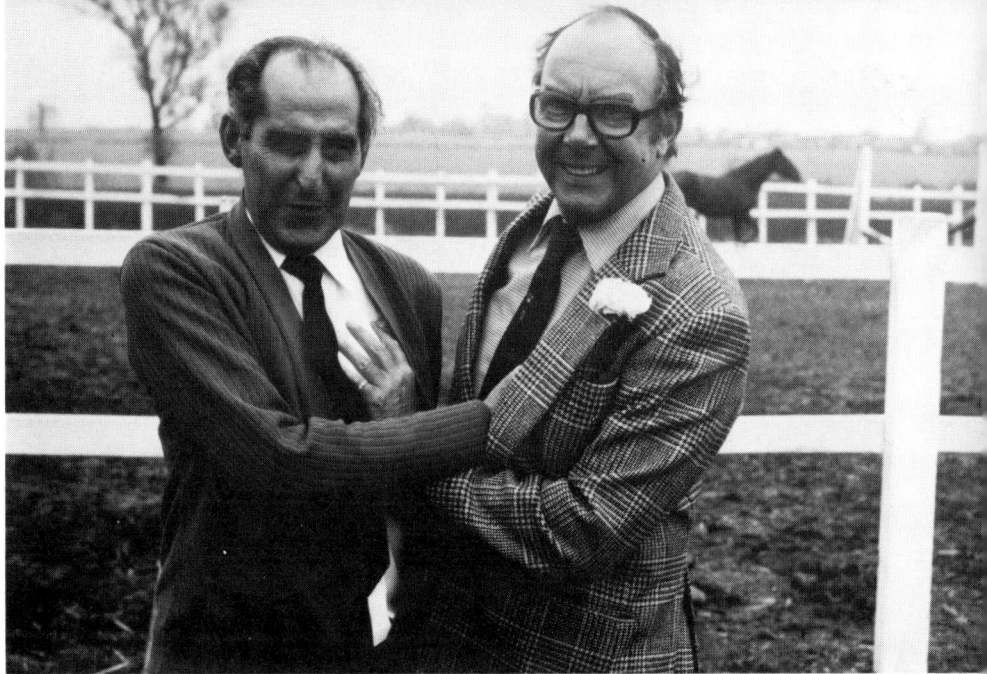

Above With Eric Morecambe at Jackie's farm in Northampton (*Evening News*).

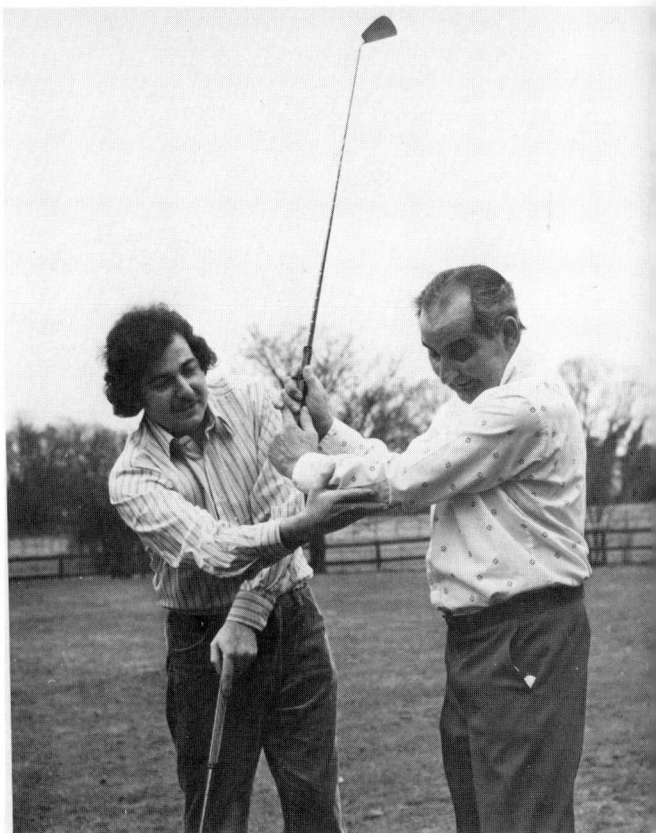

Right I had a game of golf with Andrew Barlow on the day he was discharged from Papworth (*Daily Mail*).

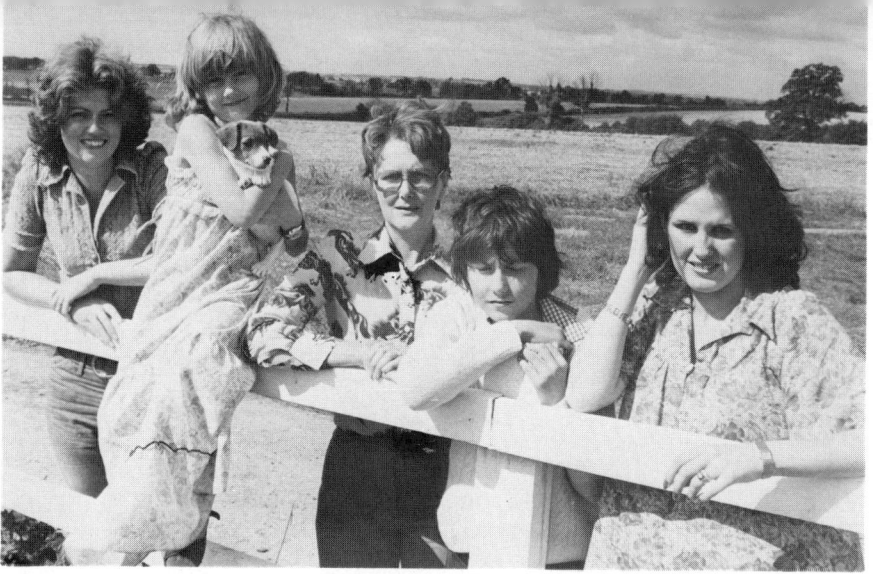
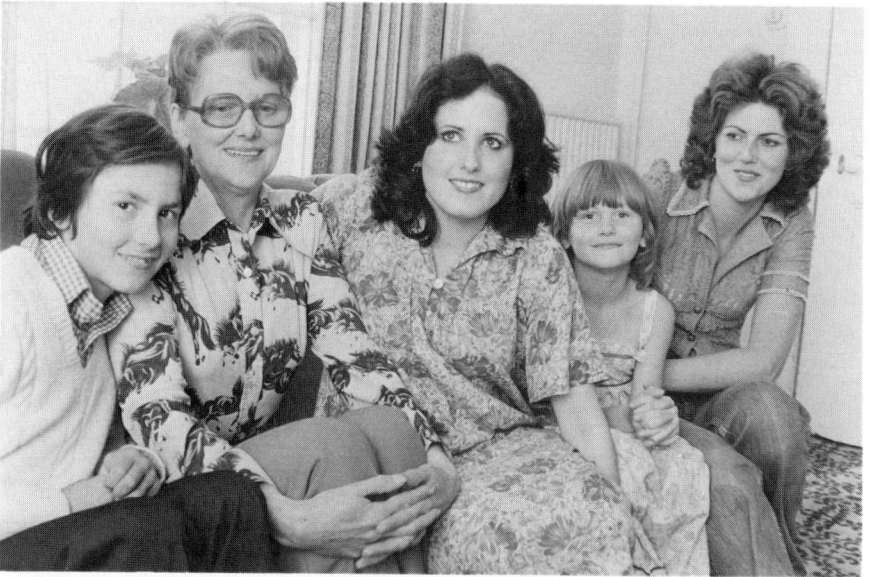
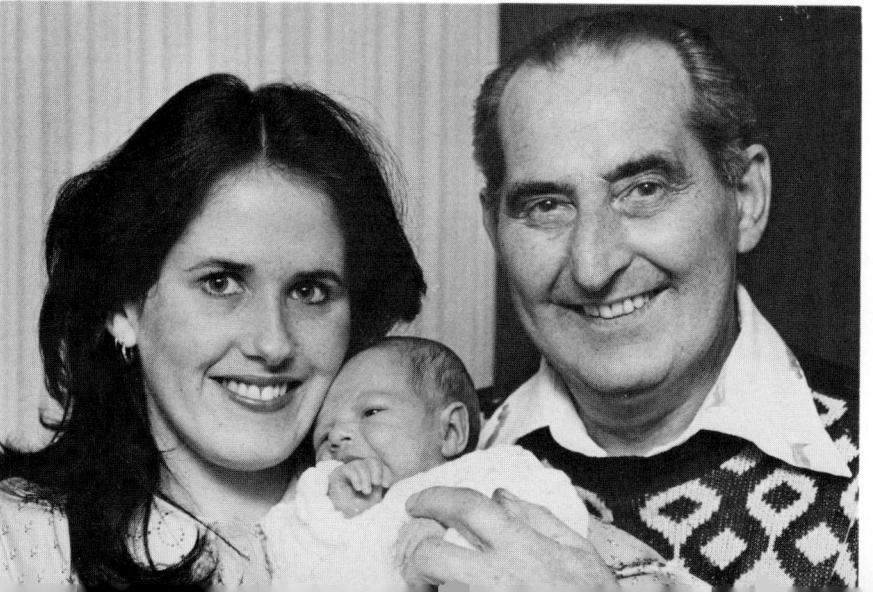

Left Jackie, Samantha (and Peanuts), Doreen, Kevin and Wendy at the farm *(The Northampton Chronical & Echo)*.

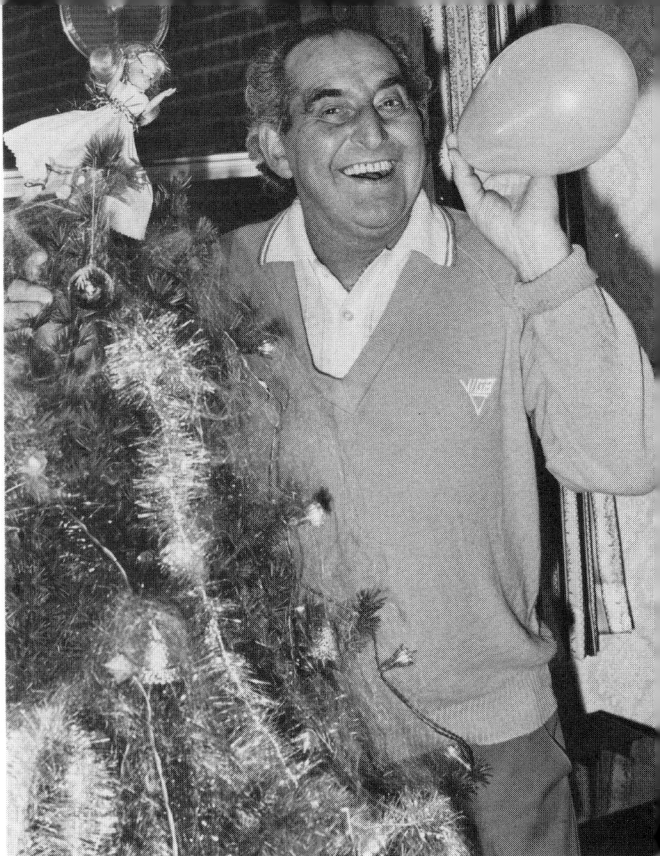

Centre left Kevin, Doreen, Wendy, Samantha and Jackie at the farm *(The Northampton Chronicle & Echo)*.

Bottom left With Wendy and my grand-daughter, Alexandra. I was so happy that baby Alex was born in St George's *(Evening News)*.

Above right Christmas 1981 *(Express Newspapers)*.

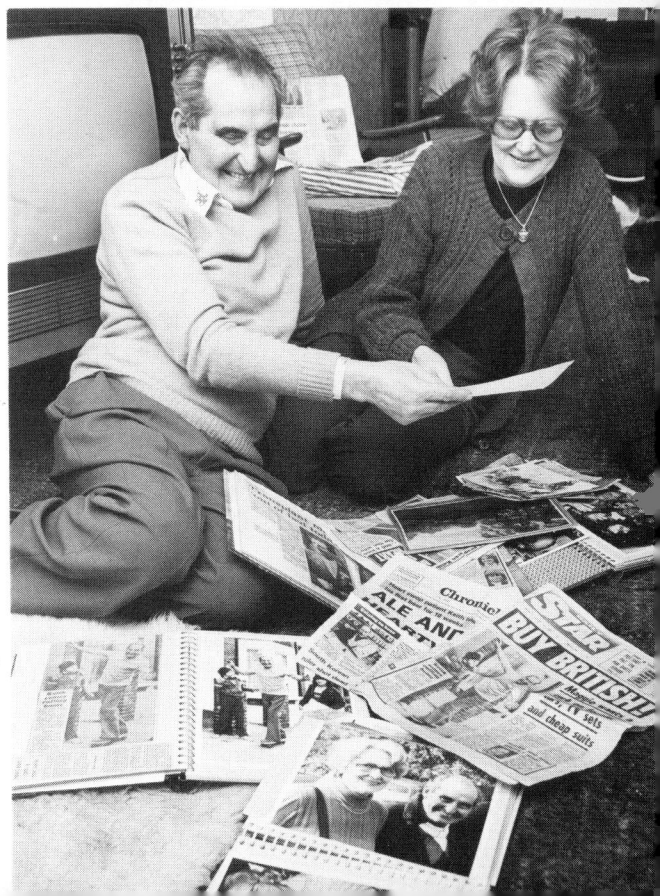

Right Looking at our many press cuttings *(Express Newspapers)*.

Overleaf My second grand-daughter, baby Alexandra *(Reginald Burkett, Express Newspapers)*.

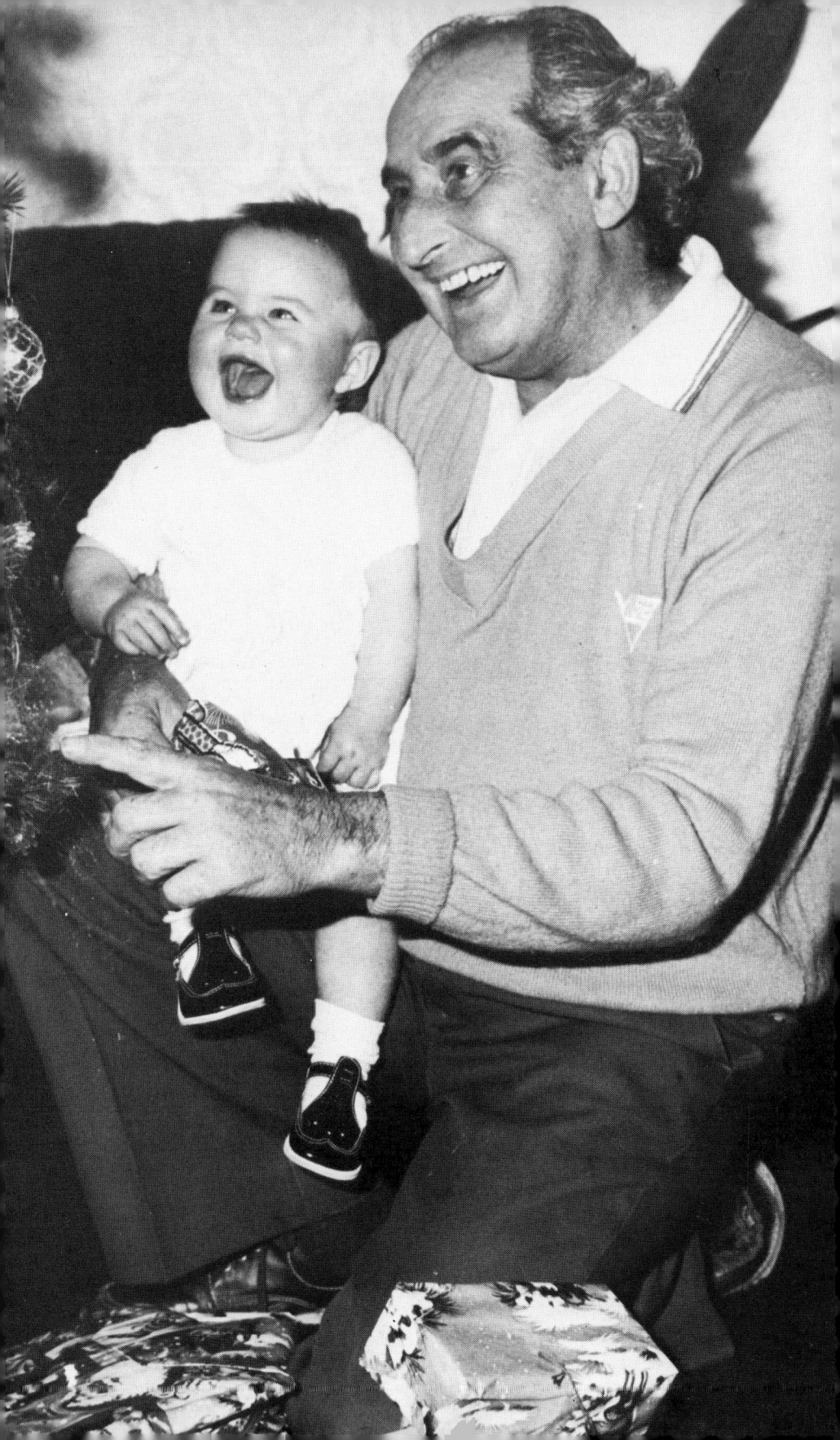

Clapham Junction!) so that he could choose the easiest way to whatever part of the heart he wanted to get at. On one occasion he thought he had found an easier route, and instead of going in through the jugular vein he went in through a vein on the left-hand side of me. He explained what he was doing, but it turned out to be a non event. He couldn't quite bend the wires enough to go through one little section, so we had to abandon that route. He apologised and went back to the jugular vein. It was OK with me. Anyhow, with his marvellous unflappable nature, a patient had to be at ease.

By now, mail was coming into my room in vast quantities. There were letters from well-wishers from all over the place. I'd go through the letters with the nurse on duty and we would read the nice things that people said. There was only one really nasty letter—from some hippy-type people from North London. I forget the actual wording, but it was to the effect that now the fuzz had got my heart I couldn't run away. It upset me and Broughie said: 'Don't upset youself, Keith, people like that are not worth bothering about.' 'I'm not upset in that way,' I replied, 'I'd just like to throttle them for sending me a letter like that.' The only other letter which brought tears to my eyes was from the current owner of our dog, Lady. At one stage of my illness, Lady had literally become too much for me. Being a boisterous Jack Russell, she used to drag me up the street far faster than I could possibly walk, so she had to go. We wanted to find her a good home and a couple in Northampton, who had heard the story from my Jackie, took Lady on. Anyhow, when I had this nice letter telling me all about Lady, I literally had tears in my eyes. It was amazing that some of the mail arrived at all—some letters were addressed simply to 'The Heart Man, Cambridge' or even 'The Heart Man, England'. They were all delivered and some of them had notes from the postmen on the back, wishing me well.

One of the nicest pieces of mail I received was a telegram from Eric Morecambe extolling the virtues of his team, Luton, and blaming the fact that I was a Fulham supporter for my landing in Papworth! I sent him a ribald one back, but I think it got watered down a little bit!

The newspapers were another story. Like everything else, including the letters, anything which came into the room had to be autoclaved. This was OK for the letters inside envelopes, but the newspapers used to arrive like pieces of toast—baked brown and stiff. I told the nurses that, in the old days, when a woman was in labour, the midwife used to grab newspapers and lay them on the floor as they were so sterile, so why did they have to be baked in this day and age? They carried out some tests in the lab and eventually I got newspapers which had been sprayed with a chemical, so I was at least able to have the papers first thing in the morning, instead of baked brown, last thing at night.

When Jackie heard this, she said she would bring in all the Press cuttings for me. 'What Press cuttings?' I asked. I hadn't taken too much notice of these, except the solomn pronouncements which Mr English had made. She said: 'Good gracious, Dad—you've been in the headlines!' 'You're joking!' I exclaimed. 'I thought there might be a couple of lines in the local rag, but national headlines—no!' Up until that stage, it really and truthfully hadn't registered with me. When eventually Jackie did bring in the cuttings, it took me a couple of days to read them all and I just couldn't believe what they said. Because of the sensible way in which the operation had been talked about, I just took it as a routine job!

The first letter I wrote was to Harry Lowe. I knew how he felt. I don't suppose anyone else in the world realised his feelings, but I did. I had a wonderful letter back from him, full of congratulations, but Harry must have been wondering when his turn was going to come.

The volume of congratulatory mail was growing and I distinctly remember, on that horrific day when Lord Louis Mountbatten was blown up, that there were some marvellous letters from people in Ireland, and I still get letters from people all over the place and even now from Ireland, despite all their troubles. The nicest part of receiving all this mail were the letters renewing old friendships from schoolboy days and service days.

One day, a letter arrived with the post mark 'Reading'. Without looking for a sender's address on the back, I knew who it was from— Dickie Christie, an old friend of mine. Sure enough it was, but the most tragic part about it is, because all these hundreds of letters couldn't stay in the ward, Doreen used to take them back to the farm. In doing so, we lost Dickie's address, and I haven't had a chance to trace him since. So, if you read this, Dickie, do get in touch.

There were also many telephone calls. Some of them were from people claiming to know me but in fact they didn't and, in the end, the calls were vetted so as to give me some peace. One day, John Edwards came in to ask me if I knew a chap called Steve Nash, who sounded very genuine. 'Yes,' I replied, 'he's an old school friend.' Apparently Steve had said to John that he realised I would be up to my neck in calls and letters, but that he would be quite willing to wait a few months to hear from me and would leave his telephone number. I was delighted to make contact with him after I came out of Papworth. It turns out that now he is a big wheel in the oil industry.

By now, I had started to reply to correspondence sent to me. I started a routine that I have continued to this day. That is to deal with letters from anyone awaiting surgery or who has a heart problem first and foremost—I put them on the top of my list. Consequently, unfortunately, the backlog of my mail has now got out of hand. I would like to take this opportunity now to say to anyone who has written to me and hasn't had an answer, please accept my deepest apologies, but I just cannot keep up. I am sure you all know how much your letters mean to me.

Life in the 'bubble' carried on routinely for the next couple of weeks. I woke up early and washed myself. After this I changed the bed linen and cleaned the room. Dirty linen was thrown through the sliding door for the laundry. Observations were carried out on my by the duty nurse, dressings were changed and ECGs carried out. The duty surgeon would come in and take any blood samples required and if he couldn't do it, Ray Latimer, the Consultant Anaesthetist would do it. After this, breakfast.

Throughout the day there would be other observations to make, or possibly a visit from Mr English, but, other than that, the day was more or less mine. The only change was that I was now showing the first side effects of the steroids I was taking. In my case it was mouth herpes so I had some rather unpleasant ulcers. These ulcers were to plague me for several months—for at least six months even after I was discharged from Papworth.

By this time, Doreen had brought me in some watercolour paper and watercolour paints—nothing very elaborate because it had to be autoclaved through and she couldn't bring tubes of paint in for fear of them exploding during this process. However, I had a palette type set of paints and I started amusing myself doing some watercolours, because painting was my first love. They didn't turn out very well because of the paints which I was using, but I thoroughly enjoyed doing it. I had also struck up a friendship with a squirrel outside my room. A bit of a long-distance friendship, I'll grant you. The squirrels used to leap about in the trees, but this one used to sit on a wall, a storey lower than me and at least 20 feet out, but it would sit there and stare at my window for hours on end, and I used to stare back at it, because I was so fascinated by it. One day, one of the nurses, seeing me staring vacuously into space, tapped on my window and asked if I was OK. She thought I might have been depressed, but I quickly explained that I was concentrating on this squirrel and could have watched it for hour after hour. I had heaps of time.

I stayed in the Barrier Room for eight weeks and, apart from the routine checks and other things, night became day and day night. I had my share of sleep whenever I wanted to, so if I wanted to get up in the night to do some painting, the nurses let me get on with it, knowing I would sleep during the day.

During the course of one evening, I felt slightly sore inside, following another biopsy. I took no notice of it. As usual, round about 2 o'clock in the morning, I got out of bed and started to do some watercolouring. Sister Chris was on night duty at the time, and came in to have a casual chat with me. In the course of conversation I told her I was a bit sore after this biopsy, where I hadn't been with any of the others. 'Don't worry,' she said sympathetically, 'you must remember the wires are going down the same route all the time and now and then you're bound to get a little internal soreness.' 'Oh yes, I appreciate that,' I answered, 'but the funny part is I am so short of breath as well.' She asked me to repeat what I had just said. When I did, she surprised me by telling me to get on my bed straight away. 'Don't clown about, Chris.' I argued. 'Will you please get on that bed straight away,' she ordered. Something in the tone of her voice made me realise that she really meant what she said and I obliged. She wouldn't even let me clean up my watercolours.

She called the duty surgeon who took one look at me and sent for the X-ray machine. Now this was a bit awkward, because every time they brought the machine into the Barrier Room it had to be thoroughly washed and sterilised. It caused a lot of work and sometimes afterwards the machine had to be stripped completely due to the water getting in. Anyway, eventually it arrived and after examining the plates it became evident that my lung had collapsed as a result of that morning's biopsy. It was Andrew Thorpe who had then to insert a tube into my side to blow my lung up again and it was Woggie and Avril who subsequently removed it. But it wasn't as straightforward as that.

I don't know if the procedure of the insertion and removal of this tube carried out on me was the norm, but there was a good deal of joking between me and my doctors and I was quite happy with the proceedings. Andrew made a little mark between my ribs, gave it a little local anaesthetic and made a puncture mark on the flesh and he was casually talking to me as he held the plastic tube in line with the incision that he had made. Whilst he was doing this he said: 'Are you prepared for what I'm going to do?' No sooner than I had got the word, 'Yes', out of my mouth he whopped the other end with his hand and forced the tube through the incision in my skin and into my lung. It was a bit of a surprise, as I thought it was a bit primitive, but if that was a surprise, it was nothing compared to the way in which Woggie removed it after my lung had blown up. He got some strong surgical line and tied it around this plastic tube. He twisted this like a fisherman's twist and Avril wrapped it round her hands. She then put her knee against my chest, which to me could only imply a great heaving action. Whilst Woggie was cutting a couple of stiches which were holding the tube in position, he said to me: 'When I say "go" Keith, I want you to take a deep breath in and wriggle like ***!' It was most probably the only time I have ever heard Woggie use an expletive. Anyhow, Woggie yelled:

'Go!' I took a breath and wriggled like frenzy. Avril pushed with her knee and pulled with her arms and, with one almighty heave, out popped the tube and it was all over.

When he heard about it, Dr Petch came and apologised about the biopsy but he was grinning all over his face as he knew well that I didn't take a blind bit of notice of having my lung inflated—just as long as it had the necessary effect.

During the tail end of the first week after the operation, Mr Edwards had allowed the Press agencies to send a representative photographer to take pictures of me in the 'bubble', also a photographer representing the evening newspapers. By now the Press were clamouring for a bit more information, not just general hand-outs. Naturally, all the newspapers wanted an exclusive story. The decision was ours—who should we give it to? All the family were giving Doreen different advice as to which paper to choose and she got well and truly flustered and came to ask my opinion. I told her not to take any notice of anybody and that I would leave it to her to make up her own mind. I swear that Doreen settled on *The Daily Mail* for no other reason than this: she felt very sorry for the young reporter, who was sitting huddled up in a freezing car, trying to get a story. When I told John Edwards her reasons for choosing this particular paper, he almost tore his hair out! Doreen had fallen for the oldest ploy in the book. So what—what did it matter, it had to be one or other of them.

Eventually, Linda Lee Potter arrived at Papworth to do the story. Now poor old John was determined to be seen as impartial and not to show any favouritism to any one paper. As far as he was concerned the paper had been chosen, but they were not going to get the privilege of photographing any hospital equipment. To be honest, he was a bloody nuisance at that time. We even had to cover up the brand name on the bike pedalling machine so the company wouldn't benefit from the publicity. All the time the poor girl was doing her interview, John would pop in and out, checking whether I was too tired to carry on. This must have thoroughly distracted her attention, and how she ever got a story out of it is a mystery to me. Still, John was doing his job and he always did that properly.

One good thing came out of this interview. Up to then the children (Kevin and my grand-daughter, Samantha) were only allowed into the room on a few special visits, but after the newspaper interview, they now became regular visitors. The other major event at that time was that, just prior to the interview, the last remaining lines attaching me to machines had been removed. Just before they removed them, the drug dispensing line started leaking. They repaired this, but soon the small leak spread into a split in the lead. Repairs were ineffectual so there were two choices—either put a replacement lead in or do away with the machine altogether. Mr English explained that they were now almost at the end of the heavy drug dispensation so they might as well take the line out. If all was well after that, any drugs I needed would have to be administered by injection. It was a real treat to be free of this line and, psychologically, it did me a lot of good because now, for the first time, I was not attached to any sort of life support machine. I was on my own once again.

The nursing routine for the Barrier Room had also been altered. From now on the strict scrubbing and protective regulations were relaxed. Visitors now only had to put on overshoes, a gown and wear a mask. The same went for me when I left the room. When I went out for walks in the corridors, or around the duckpond, all I had to wear were overshoes and a mask. I felt well on the way to recovery. The next decision to be made was to transfer me from the 'bubble' to the other end of the ward. Unfortunately, when they wanted to move me originally a patient had developed a leg infection and they decided not to take any chances. On another occasion when they were going to move me they weren't able to as another patient had a chest infection. At least I was able to walk up the corridor to the loo now, instead of using the commode, and the physiotherapist used to take me out twice a day for exercise around the duckpond—that was more than enough for me. I loved those journeys round the duckpond, because all the cardiac patients who were sitting out on the balconies used to wave and shout out good luck messages. It was a very happy period. Unfortunately I was still plagued with the herpes. Eating things like toast really aggravated the ulcers and made it most unpleasant for me so Mr English decided that I needed some new teeth.

A dental surgeon from Addenbrooke's visited me in the 'bubble' and took a plaster cast, then went away to make me some teeth. He didn't return to Papworth with them himself because he was busy, so he sent them for me to try. If they fitted, all well and good; if they didn't I was to let him know and at the first available opportunity he was to come down and see what was wrong. Possibly he realised that they wouldn't work out very well anyway because the shape of my mouth was altering every day due to my problems with the ulcers. Consequently, I used to keep a little sharp knife and used to shave off the offending part of the teeth where they aggravated the ulcer of the day! Avril used to do her nut when she saw me filing away and eventually threatened to report me to the surgeons. It took a lot of discipline on my part to get used to semi-dentures as they did press on my ulcers and hurt me a lot.

Everything seemed to be going swimmingly until just before the fifth week and then, wham—*rejection*! Mr English and the whole team were fairly dejected at this time because it was the first real setback they had had so far. He tried Methyl Prednisolone to cure the rejection but this

94

failed and so he arranged for a special drug to be flown in from America. Soon after its arrival at Papworth, Mr English came to my room to explain that he had to go away for a few days. He also told me that he had been told by Stamford Hospital in California that the drug caused excruciating pain but there was nothing he could do other than offer me pain killers and arrange that hot towels would be available to wrap around my limbs should the pain be bad. There would be a course of four injections, with one per day.

Mr English gave me the first one himself, just before he went away. It was an intra-muscular injection into my left thigh. (The second injection was in my big toe on the left foot, the third was in my right thigh and the fourth was in my big toe on the right foot.) After Mr English had given me the first injection, he stood back waiting for the pain to occur, but nothing happened. He came back an hour later, just prior to his departure, to ask if I felt any discomfort at all. I replied that I felt fine. In fact it seemed like a let down to me, as I had braced myself for a lot of pain. However, about three hours later, I began to feel a little throbbing in my leg. Six hours later, it was far from throbbing and was giving me hell but, after nine hours, it was a shocking pain. It was the type of pain you get with a very badly pulled muscle, but it was continuous and exceedingly hard to bear. Of course, the next day, when I had the next injection, it was in the big toe of the *same* leg, so it doubled the strength of the pain I already had. The peculiar thing was that, after they had finished the full course, the right leg was two days behind the left leg (as far as the pain went) but it recovered more quickly than the left leg. I am sure that this course of treatment has permanently weakened my legs a little bit. I may be stupid, but I am one of those people who don't like taking pills, and for the next few days I suffered really bad pain and the nurses used to say to me: 'Don't be an idiot, Keith, why don't you take some painkillers?' But I said I'd rather have the pain than take painkillers unnecessarily—but it was a close run thing.

Afterwards, when Andrew Barlow (who followed me into the 'bubble') had his rejection, he was also given this drug although his course was administered in a slightly different way. The pain hit him immediately. Anyway, we are the only two people to have had the treatment in this way and from then on it has been given through a drip. I also believe that, in America (where this drug was the standard form of treatment and where it was given in the muscle), the nurses may have squirted a little of the drug on the floor before injecting, only to cause a little less pain to their patients. But as far as TE was concerned, drugs had to be administered in the proper dosage.

Years later, when I was on the platform at the Royal Festival Hall, addressing the nurses at the International Convention of Intensive

Care, I was involved in a question and answer session and the subject of this drug came up. I told a nurse from Stamford Hospital that I was prepared to have this treatment again and again, if needs be. I explained that I considered myself lucky to have had the drug available to me and that to this day, I haven't even had a hint of rejection. However, I must emphasise that this treatment is now no longer used.

The question of drugs for heart transplant patients was naturally one of the main things I discussed with Emmanuel Vitrai much later. (For those of you who don't know, he is the *world's* longest surviving heart transplant patient. His operation was 13 years ago!) Doreen had mentioned to a newspaper reporter that we would like to meet Emmanuel. As this would make a nice story, the Editor, much to our amazement, arranged for Doreen and me to go to Marseilles where Emmanuel lived. We had a marvellous two-day trip which was very interesting. I found out that Emmanuel was on the earlier types of drugs which were in use at the time of his operation. He now has to inject himself *three* times a day. He calls himself 'The World's Most Injected Man!' He couldn't believe it when I told him that I only had to take a few pills. He then asked me for my surgeon's name and the address of Papworth Hospital in order to see if he could get a prescription for the pills instead of having injections. You see, poor old Emmanuel is in a bit of a spot. All the surgeons who operated on him have subsequently died of heart attacks! I told him I thought he would be mad to change horses in midstream, having gone along for so long with a method which obviously suited him well. I'm still in favour of sticking to the drugs which I have tried and tested and which have worked, even though new drugs are always being introduced. The only side effect I have experienced with my drugs is putting on a bit of weight—personally I'd rather be fat and alive, than skinny and dead! I, for one, was quite happy with what I was on and I still am.

Anyway, back to the story at Papworth. At that time, Doreen stopped visiting me at weekends. This was in order to give her a little break from the week's visits and give the family and friends who came up from London or elsewhere a chance to see me. It was amusing that sometimes she had to draw up a rota of visitors! I also had other visitors who lived nearby but who had not visited me before because of the strict routine in the 'bubble'. These included Dr Smailes and his wife, other friends who had been in Papworth and had been discharged and even Alma who, up until then, had only waved and chatted to me through the glass. Now all she needed to do was put on her mask and overshoes and it was simple.

One of the nicest visitors was Mrs Burnett (Chairman of the Cambridge Area Health Authority.) She had made my operation possible. Apparently, the National Health Service had given Papworth Hospital the money for two heart transplant operations. The first operation on Charlie McHugh was not a success. There was, therefore, only enough money in the kitty for one more operation. I understand that many people from the health authority wanted to put a stop to this operation and it was Mrs Burnett's strength of character and courage which made them change their minds. She, alone, was responsible for Mr English having the second crack of the whip. Because of this, the second operation *had* to succeed otherwise there would have been no future operations. I have often been tempted to ask Mr English: 'Why me? Why me?' It is a question that Doreen and I have often burned to ask. Still, it was Mrs Burnett's persistence which enabled me to have my transplant. I was so pleased for her (and for me) that it worked out fine for everybody. If anything had gone wrong, I would hardly have known about it, but it might have affected the transplant programme for many years to come.

I had asked Mr English soon after my operation if I could write to thank Mrs Burnett. I didn't pretty the letter up with little phrases, I just thanked her and told her how much I admired her guts, so it was so nice that she came to visit me. I know she was thrilled as well—maybe she was also a bit relieved that her efforts had been justified. (Later, when we started to form the Papworth Hospital Transplant Club, I put forward her name to be on our Board, and I'm very glad to say that she accepted.)

There was still quite a lot of security at this time to prevent the Press from getting into the hospital grounds and here is a little story which may amuse you. One night, quite late, my son, Keith, and a few of his friends drove up to visit me. Papworth didn't mind Keith visiting me late at night because they realised that he had to come up from London. I was allowed out into a little hall to chat with Keith and company. All of a sudden, one of the nurses who had been warned to watch out for the Press, came rushing up and said: 'Keith, you're sure these gentlemen aren't Press, aren't you?' We all looked at each other and burst out laughing. 'Love,' I said, 'between the lot of them they'd have difficulty in spelling CAT'. That put her mind at rest, but John Edwards then issued a notice that there would be no more bulletins to the Press until the day of my release. John and I did discuss what would happen when I was discharged, but I wish he had warned me just how much pressure there would be. However, I think he knew that I would not be a patsy and I certainly wasn't a get-rich-quick merchant.

By this time, I was able to get better paints into the Barrier Room as they had started spraying them with antiseptics and had found that this worked. This meant that not everything had to be autoclaved so at last I had some oil paints and canvasses—far nicer than the little water colours

97

that I had been using up to then. I feverishly used to try to keep down the smell of turps in the room in case Mr English had any objections, but he didn't ever comment on it. I tried to keep as much paint off my hands as possible, too, as I wasn't sure what effect it would have on my germ-free existence at that stage.

There was now a lot of talk about moving me out of the Intensive Care Unit and transferring me to the top floor of the hospital. This was to enable me to have a less 'barriered' existence and to give me more freedom. In other words, when I got to that room, I could more or less mingle with the other patients up there. Eventually the move was made but, as my room wasn't ready immediately, I was put temporarily into a two-bedded ward instead. Alma and another nurse had carried out a strict barrier procedure on the room, trying to make it as germ-proof as possible. They set about sticking brown paper over the joints of the windows, but Alma was extremely worried about the top pane which was broken, and she didn't know what to do about it! When she pointed it out to Mr English he replied that I didn't need my windows sealed any more and could open them now if I wished. As soon as I heard that, the windows were literally flung wide open! It was lovely to have fresh air into the ward at last.

None of the nurses on the top floor had had any experience of tending to a heart transplant patient so this was going to be a new experience for them. They were all on tenterhooks and took great care to look after me. There was an observation window in the door of the room but, unfortunately for nurse Ophelia, the window was still 3 inches above the top of her head! I used to roll with laughter when I saw this little head bobbing up and down as she jumped up to see if I was OK. She soon found herself a small pair of platform steps and used these when she came to have a look at me.

Now, I shall tell you how Alma was a wee bit naughty, and bent a couple of rules for me. Outside the room which I was to have was a marvellous beech tree but, unfortunately, it obscured most of the view of the pond and some lovely buildings which I wanted to paint, so she asked the patient next door to swop with me and he did. I then had an uninterrupted view of the area I wanted to paint! The other gentleman didn't mind at all—the rooms themselves were identical and he wasn't interested in painting!

When I at last got into my single room, it was nurse Jeanie's turn to worry (she was a night auxiliary). As this particular room didn't have a glass observation panel in the door, she had to open my door to see how I was. I used to make her anxious as I was often flat out, sleeping soundly, not moving a muscle and it wasn't until she came right up to me that she could tell whether or not I was dead or alive! Eventually, when the rest of the patients on the top floor had settled, I used to prop my door open about 18 inches, and leave my curtain around my bed slightly open, so Jeanie could pop her head around the door when she liked.

Now I was allowed to mix with the other patients but, having been in the Barrier Room for eight weeks, I had become used to my own company. At last I had what I had always wanted—a room of my own where I could paint quietly. Mr English was a little concerned that I was keeping myself to myself and gently hinted that I should mingle with the other patients a little more, which for his sake, I did. There were a few occasions when I would be warned not to go to certain parts of the hospital because of a patient with some sort of infection—I still had to be careful about this risk.

When I eventually got out of the Intensive Care Unit and on to the top floor, one of my first visitors was Percy, my friend from St George's. I'm sure he came to run his eagle eye over the place, as well as visit me, in case he ended up having a transplant himself! Old Percy doesn't leave anything to chance. Still, Percy and I managed to break the rules as usual. It was a boiling hot day and Perce was sweating profusely under his mask. I told him not to worry and to let the damned thing dangle in front of his face—I didn't think it mattered as long as we were far apart from each other. Of course, who should walk into the room but Dr Petch—the very man who Percy would have to go to for assessment should he want a transplant! He looked in horror at Percy lounging about in a very unhygienic state. Well, quite naturally, Percy and I had some good laughs during that visit. He also told me about all the goings-on in Harris Ward, giving me messages from everyone, including love from all the girls, which I sent back. (They had all written marvellous letters to me. I had heard from Celia who had been transferred to John Radcliffe Hospital at Oxford, but the sweetest letter of the lot came from Rachael. In it she explained that she was on night duty and, at about 2 am when all was quiet, she had felt that she had to sit down and write to me. She poured out her feelings and her affections for her old patient in a lovely letter which I still treasure today.) Percy eventually left, after we had made arrangements to meet at Hyde Park Corner where I would have to go for my check-ups following my discharge from Papworth.

Dr Petch soon informed me that he had made arrangements for me to have another visitor, whom I greatly looked forward to seeing. It was Bill Ginks. He had to discuss the therapy which I was going to require when I left hospital, at Papworth and St George's alternately. After the usual enquiries, Bill told me exactly what I could and couldn't do when I left hospital. To the best of my ability, considering how much running around I do, I have stuck to his advice.

He advised me strongly not to be at everybody's beck and call when I came out, as this would be to the detriment of my health and well-being. He said he was sure I could cope with anything, 'like water off a duck's back', but he also said: 'The greatest thing you can do for your surgeons now is to be seen to be alive and to be seen to be thoroughly enjoying life.' Of course I have done a fair bit of running around since my operation but, as soon as I feel any real physical strain, I put the blocks on because I know what Bill said was true. So many people have done so much to give me a new life, also Bill is one of the men who I admire so much—he is truly dedicated to all his patients. When I tried to thank him for all that he had done for me, Bill brushed it aside, saying it was just his job.

So that was Bill's advice to me on my post-Papworth behaviour, and further advice came thick and fast because I was now approaching my discharge from hospital. Mike Petch came in to discuss my diet. He told me what sort of foods I could eat—I had already been told a bit about this by the dietician—but he added: 'Now, let's settle drink!' I assured him that he didn't have to worry on that count as I had never overdone it when drinking—I enjoyed a pint, but two was the absolute maximum that I could manage; I felt uncomfortable after that. He asked me how I would plan my drinking at a lengthy function. I said I would probably have a pint at the beginning and could spin this out for quite a long time and after that I would probably go on to vermouth and lemonade. I added that, should the function go on for very long, I would just have plain lemonade. Mike said he was well pleased with this, and was sure I would keep things under control.

Mr English's advice was: 'When you get out, you're going to have to attend a lot of functions and, naturally, you will go and visit friends. I know how difficult it is to take low fat margarines and powdered milks and things like that to friends and you won't know how a meal has been prepared at a function—so all I can say is, when you get home, compensate.' In other words, my only orders were—to use my loaf!

I couldn't really see what everybody meant when they talked about the functions which I would have to attend. What functions? At that stage I had no idea what I was in for!

The dietician gave me a little booklet of suitable diets and I was allowed to look after my own pills. To get me used to this I took them myself and logged what I had taken in a record book, instead of having them dispensed. As I had to be responsible for my pills for the rest of my life, it was a good idea to have a week's practice before I really took over. Then came the question of where I was going after I had been discharged. Was I returning to London or going to stay for a time with Jackie in Northampton? Mr English said he wasn't worried about where I went, although Northampton might be the best choice as I would have to attend a clinic at Papworth for two days a week, and it might be too long a drag up from London. However, the decision was mine. So it was agreed that I would stay with Jackie until just before Christmas and then return to London.

Mr Edwards then started preliminary talks with the Press about the coverage of my story. Unfortunately, an incident occurred about seven days before my discharge which caused a great deal of hullabaloo at Papworth. Bearing in mind that John Edwards had previously said that there would be no more stories or photographs released until the time of my discharge, it was a great surprise to me when I opened a national daily paper one morning, to find a photograph of myself strolling round the grounds of Papworth with Barbara, the physiotherapist. There was also a small write-up. I assured everybody that I had not been speaking to the Press. 'It's highly illegal, immoral or both,' I told everyone, 'how the devil they managed it, I don't know!'

Poor old Barbara was under suspicion for being in league with the Press. She had that day, gone down to the West Country for her holidays and apparently she spent the whole day answering telephone calls from Papworth regarding this leak. It turned out to be a 'snatch' picture. It seems that the photographer had been in the car park and taken a long-range shot of us. I suppose it was a bit of fuss about nothing, but I felt bad because poor Barbara had lost the first day of her holiday over it. John Edwards threatened to report the newspaper to the Press Council but it all blew over—there wasn't much we could do after the event.

During my last week at Papworth all the various members of staff came in to see me, among them were Papworth's convenor, Len Simmonds, and Charles Hubbard, the Senior Nursing Administrator. They often came in for a chin-wag. Charles is two years older than me and had been brought up in the same area, and gone to the same school as me (although we were two years apart). He may look 20 years older than me, but really it's only two! Sorry, Charles, I had to get that one in!

As the day of discharge drew nearer, Doreen started taking bits of my gear back to the farm and I prepared myself, with Mr Edwards' help, to meet the Press. I'd never had to go through anything like that in my life before, so I didn't know what it entailed.

Eventually, after 10 weeks at Papworth, the glorious morning arrived. I had my last breakfast, with the usual banter with the nurses about their spreading my margarine too thinly, and then 'goodbyes' to everyone. True to form, Mr English was absent. He *always* shunned publicity, so he made sure he wasn't going to be about that day! Up to the very last minute before I faced the Press, I still had to wear a mask. The arrangements were that one representative reporter would interview me in my room, before I had to go and face the Press photographers and television cameras. So, I still had my mask on when

Mr Edwards brought this chap into my room. After the interview Doreen and I went down to meet the television cameras. At the same time, people were loading my possessions into the car. I had 10 minutes with one channel and then 10 minutes with the opposition.

Then we went outside and met the barrage of Press cameras. As I promised, I gave Barbara a wave—she was looking out from one of the top floor windows. During the course of all the cameras snapping away, it all got a bit too much for Doreen. All of a sudden she burst into tears. I snuggled her head into my shoulder, calling her a silly lemon, and Alma comforted her too. She quickly recovered and the cameramen resumed their snapping. I don't know if John Edwards had a word about it to them afterwards but, to the full credit of all the papers concerned, not one of them printed a picture of Doreen in tears.

Then we set off in the car, out of Papworth's back entrance. The police had seen to everything and they blocked the road behind us so that we couldn't be followed by the Press. Travelling through St Neots, I had this terrible urge to eat a plum. I hadn't had any fresh fruit in the hospital, it all had to be tinned because fresh fruit was difficult to obtain absolutely germ free. However, it was October 26, and a little late in the plum season, so we didn't stop there. In fact, we did stop at the village of Brafield to call on some friends, Mary and Roy Arrowsmith. We did our weekend shopping there, picking up a nice leg of lamb for Sunday. We had a little celebration drink at *The Red Lion*, just to mark the occasion, then went on to the farm. There was a little Press coverage there. (Actually, the Independent Television reporter had asked earlier if he could finish off the story with a shot of us entering Jackie's home. We readily agreed. If the BBC had made a similar request we most certainly would have let them film us, too and, to show that there was no favouritism, my son-in-law Jimmy, rang them to explain what had happened.) Naturally, we spent the rest of the day very quietly indeed. All we did during the afternoon was to telephone a few friends to say I was out of hospital, and feeling grand!

8

Early days out

The next morning, we all got up early and I borrowed a pair of Jackie's gum boots and went for a marvellous stroll through the fields. I found it a bit heavy going, to tell the truth. It was the longest walk that I had taken up to then and the clay soil was clinging to my boots, adding a lot of weight for me to carry around. However, to me it was the start of my obligatory exercises.

Throughout the rest of the morning there was a gradual build up of Press photographers at the end of the driveway to the farm. They eventually sent a representative up to ask if I would like to meet them. Well, we didn't want to set the precedent of having them inside the house (the length of the drive was quite a useful 'no go' area and, enabled us to have a bit of privacy) so, I 'phoned our friends, Frances and Bob who ran the *White Hart* pub to ask if I could meet some members of the Press in their beer garden. They replied that they would be delighted to see me but because they were leaving for their holidays that day, asked if I could arrive as soon as possible. This caused a bit of a flurry amongst the Press because, after this news filtered back to Fleet Street, there was quite a scramble to get newsmen and cameramen up the motorway in time.

Anyway, down we went to the *White Hart* and, needless to say, instead of staying in the garden, the Press wanted to go inside so we ended up outnumbering the locals. Quite naturally the boys from the Press had to take a back seat whilst I shook hands and greeted many old friends again. Then we had the obligatory photos of Frances, Bob and myself holding up champagne glasses in celebration. 'Mine hosts' then set off on the journey to their holiday and left Bob's brother, Rex, in charge of the pub. *He* then had to face the television cameras! Quite honestly, I was quite at home with the Press. It was all pretty spontaneous—I was far more concerned about meeting members of the public. I will explain why later.

The next Monday, I was a little perturbed to see the resulting photographs which appeared in the various papers. In order to show each individual photographer's work, they asked me if I could pose in a different way with a different glass in my hand. It was quite hectic in the pub when this was going on. A glass would be thrust into my hand, the photographer would take a flash photo and the glass would be snatched away, only to be replaced by a different one and the procedure was repeated with another photographer. I must have had between eight and a dozen glasses pushed in my hand in this manner but funnily enough, I didn't manage to get a drink out of any. However, I was concerned what Papworth would think. It looked as though I was having a good, boozy session—in fact I had been quite teetotal. Dr Petch *did* make some acid enquiries when I attended my first clinic but I explained the situation and he understood.

Once we had got over the hurly burly of the Press interviews, Doreen and I thought that we could now settle down to a nice quiet life. Once again, we were proved completely wrong!

I had to get myself to Papworth twice a week to attend the clinics. Jackie would drive me to Brafield, the nearby village, and there I would get on the local double-decker bus and go 40 miles across country to be dropped off at the Caxton Gibbet roundabout where Sue, a nurse from the top floor of the hospital, would drive down to meet me and take me to Papworth. I attended the clinic and then hung about until Sue was ready to take me back to the bus stop. I would take the bus to Mary and Roy Arrowsmith's farm and Jackie would pick me up and take me back to her place. I could never work out the bus fare though—it was 41p single and 83p return! During this period, Doreen went back to London as the local council was trying to find us a house with less stairs than ours.

As far as the clinics went, my examinations were, of course, quite extensive. TE was very thorough and expressed his worry about my making such a long journey, but had he known that I spent a lot of the day hanging round for Sue in the damp weather, he would not have allowed it. Fortunately, he didn't know!

Approximately a fortnight after my release from Papworth Hospital, Jackie and Jimmy went over to the Channel Islands for the week-end for some showbiz event and this just left Doreen, me, Kevin and Sammy at the farm. We had just had a nice Sunday lunch and I was dozing in front of the fire when, suddenly, pandemonium broke out. In rushed Kevin shouting: 'Quick, Dad, you'd better come—I think me and my friend have set the barn alight!'

By the tone of his voice, I knew it must be serious and so I shot out to the barn like a bullet. The barn was very long with various different sections. Some were two-storey and others, like the hay storage area, were literally about 30 feet tall from floor to ceiling. On the upper floor of one section, Jimmy was storing some potatoes; they had bales of straw over and around them for protection. Kevin and his mate, Shaun, had set these alight and flames were roaring everywhere. The danger was that some of the flames were licking through the dividing wall at a

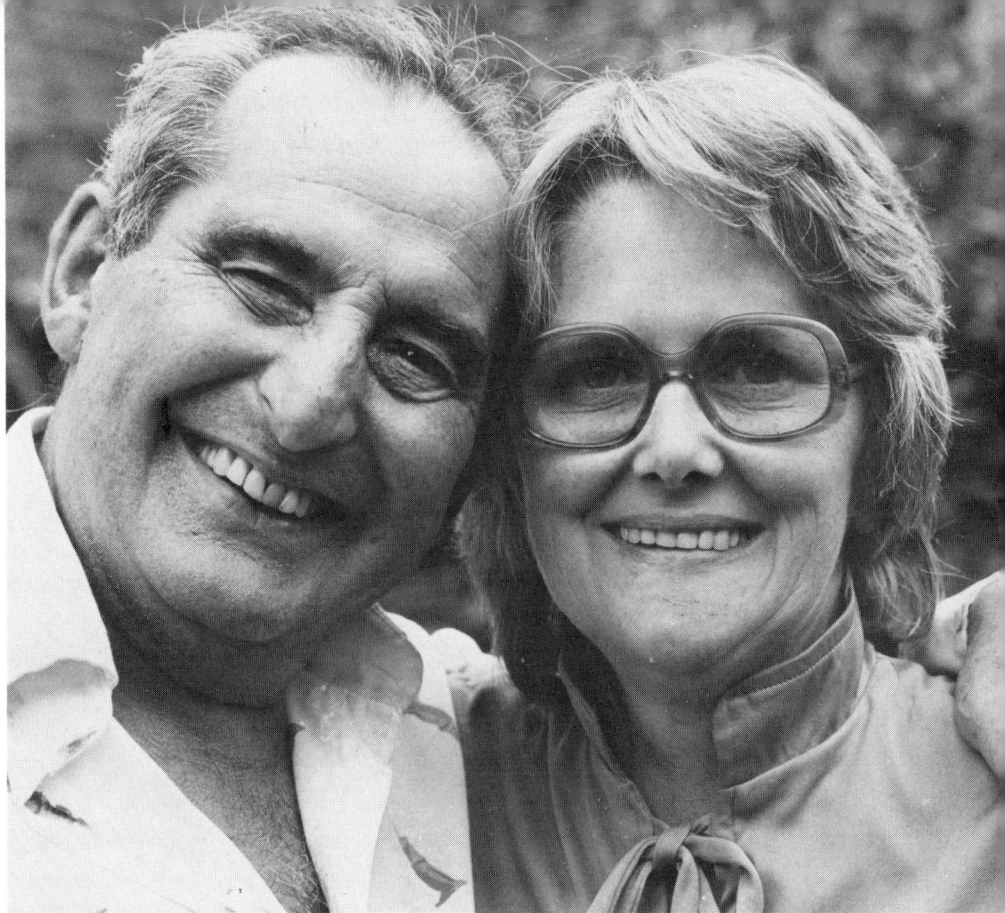

Above Doreen and me *(Express Newspapers)*. **Below** The Manulife Polo *(Manulife Ltd)*.

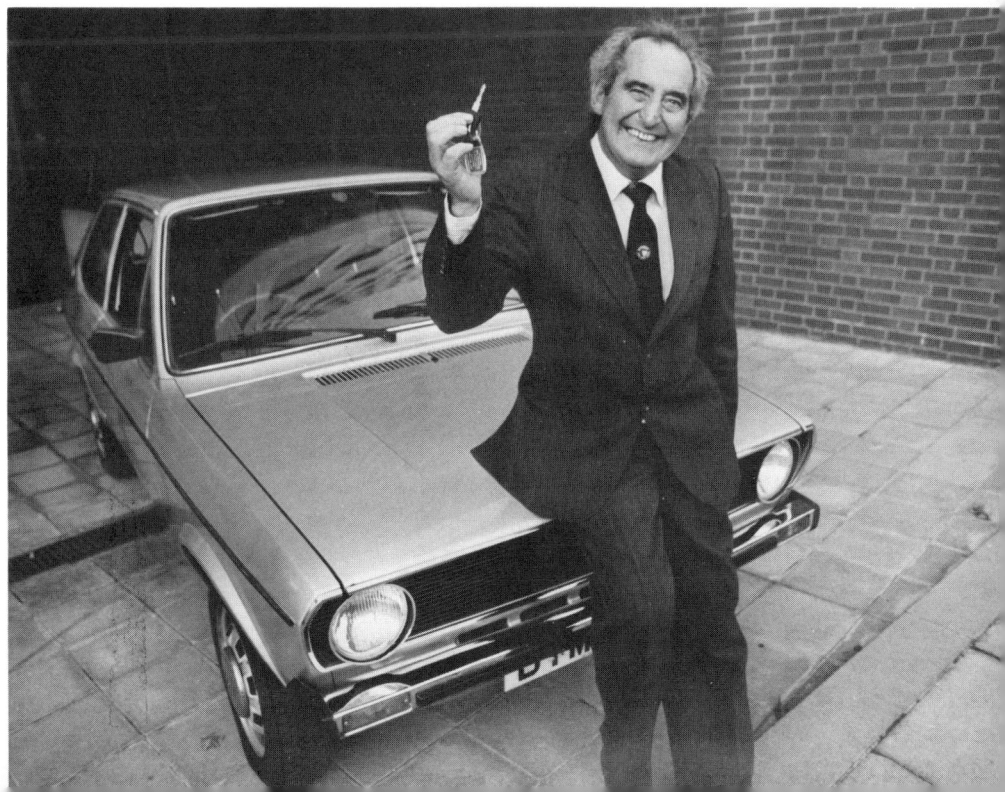

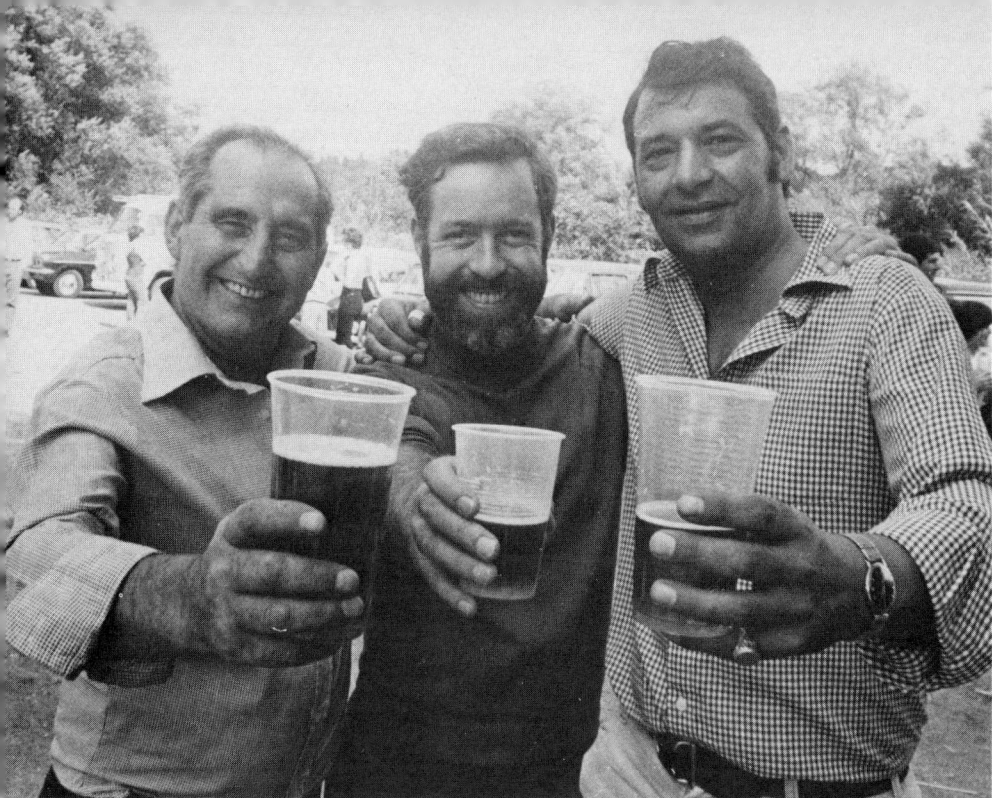

Above With the Mayor of Leighton Buzzard (centre) and Nigel Olney at Leighton Buzzard.

Below Wendy (and Alexandra), Doreen, Kevin and Keith watch me painting *(George Konig, Syndication International Ltd)*.

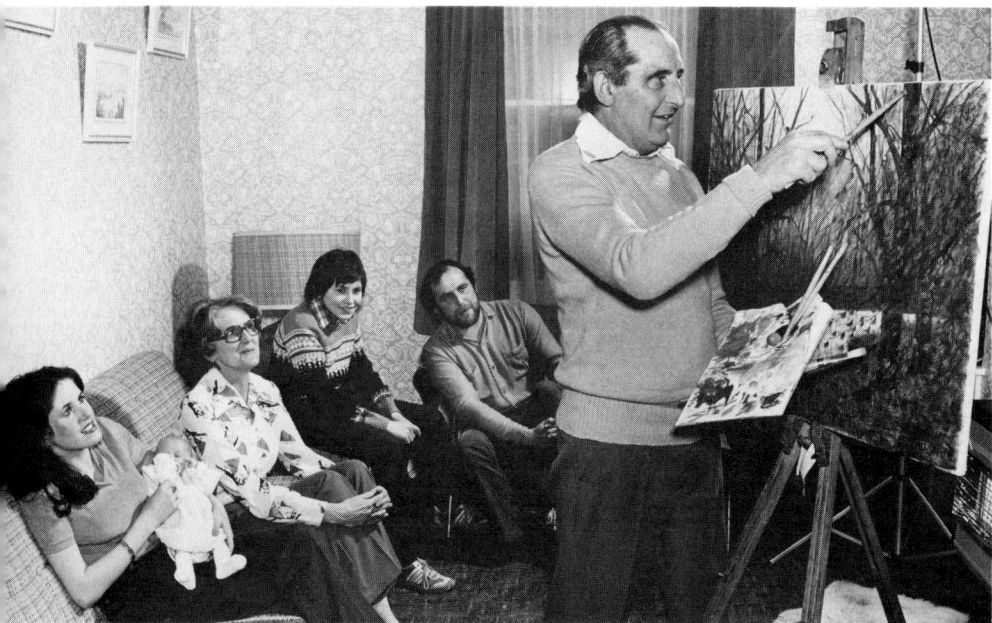

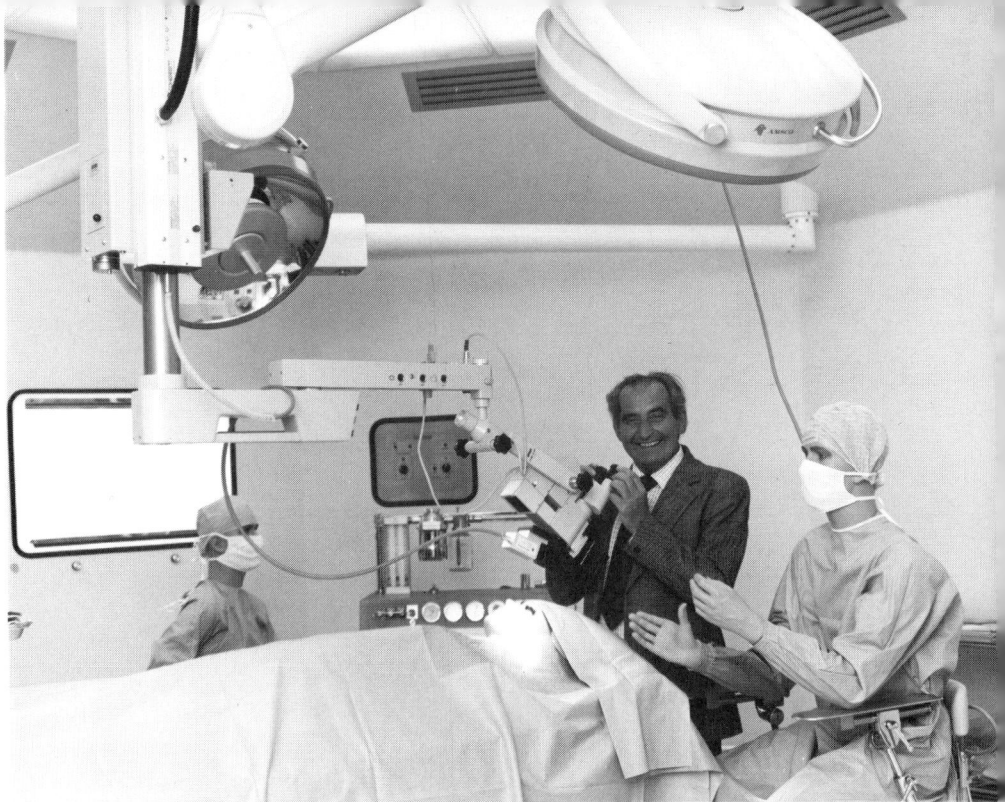

Above I opened the Medical Exhibition at Olympia in 1980 *(Pic Photos).*

Below I was delighted to meet Mrs Vera Hannant. (She had a pancreas and kidney transplant from the same donor as me.) *(Smith & Pinching Ltd, Norwich).*

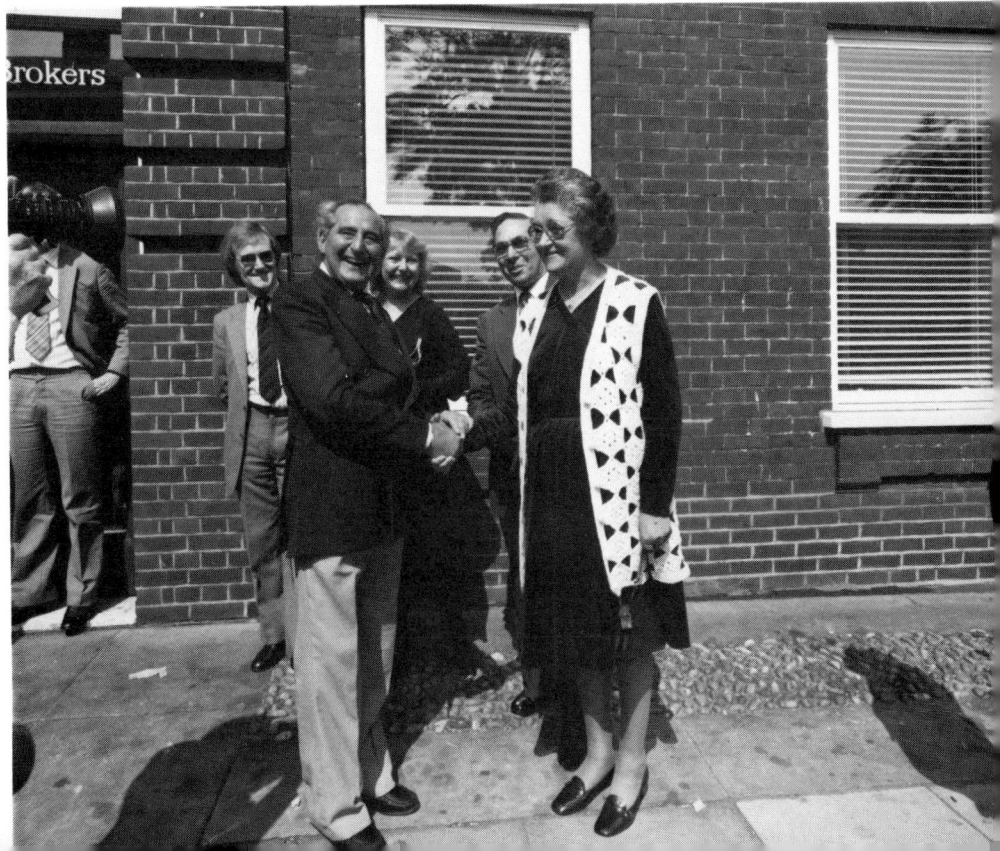

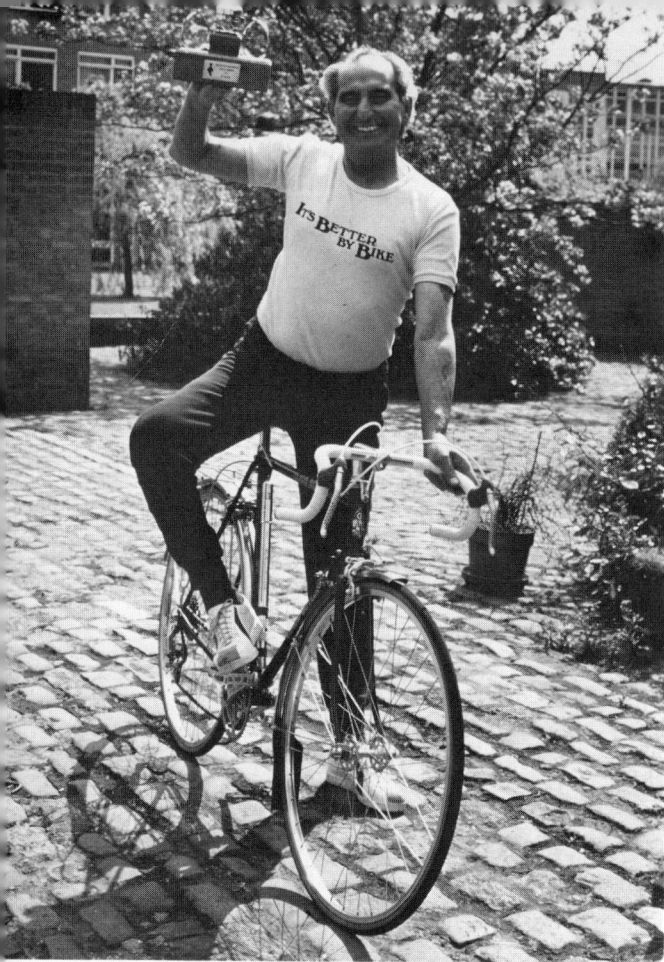

Left It's better by bike!

Below Roy Castle presenting me with the British Cycling Bureau Gold Award for Cycling.

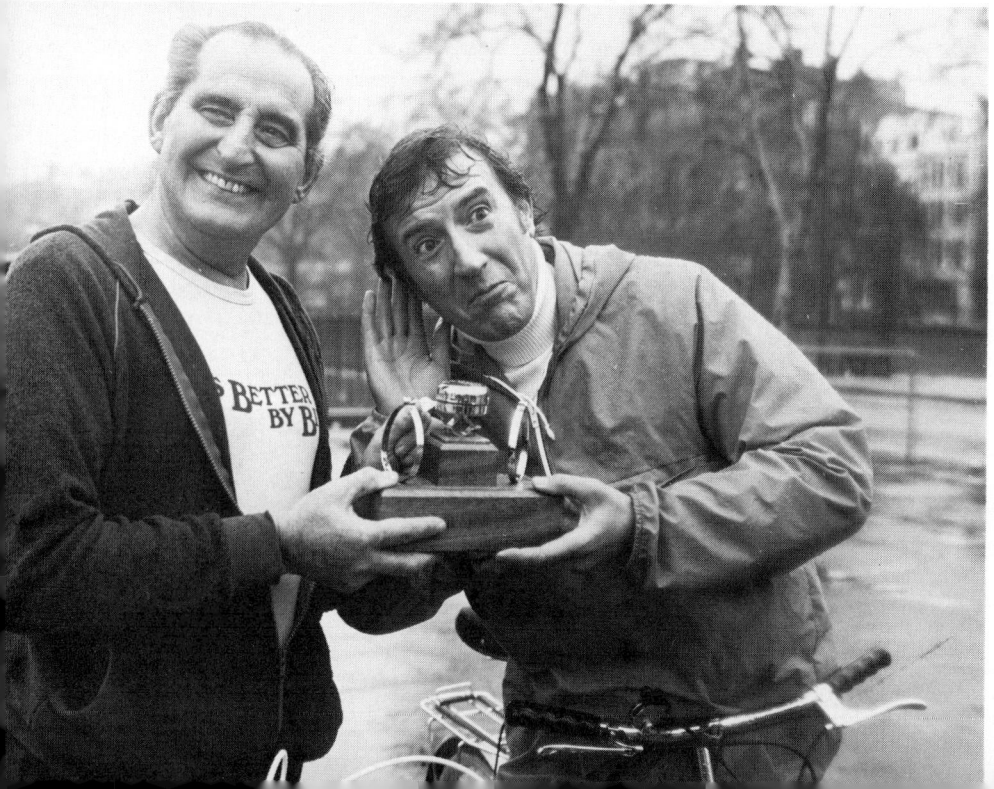

full compartment of bales of hay, 30 feet high! Within minutes the whole lot could have gone up in flames and I am talking about a building approximately 100 feet long, 30 feet wide and 30 feet high!

Well, of course we had to make a decision quickly—we were townies out in the country and the fire brigade was not within easy distance. There were horses stabled on the ground floor with some straw above them which was alight, but the real danger was that the main hay storage could quickly go up. Should we leave the horses (they weren't panicking at that time) and save the straw above, or should we get them out right away and risk the whole lot going up in flames? We opted to try to put the fire out.

By this time, the place was full of smoke and it was a question of running up the wooden stairs, taking a lungful of air, then charging into the flames, opening the upstairs doors, rushing out again to get another lungful of air, then racing back to pitch the burning straw out of the doors to the yard below. We tried to take all the straw away from the dividing wall so the main store wouldn't catch alight. The bales weighed about 60 lb—*really* good therapy for a heart transplant patient, I must say, especially bearing in mind I had orders not to scratch or cut myself!

Poor old Doreen at this time was trying to keep the horses quiet and, at the same time, trying to get extra pressure from the rather feeble hose pipe she had managed to find. In addition to the weak water pressure, the horses milling about kept treading on the hose and puncturing it. There was poor Doreen, tears in her eyes, trying to nudge the horses to one side and trying to stand on the little fountains of water, leaking out of the hose. So there she was, standing like Marilyn Monroe with her skirt blowing up in the air. There was a subtle difference—Doreen, with wet tears rolling down her cheeks and little fountains of water spurting up her kilt, wasn't exactly giving a dry laugh!

This Casey's Court atmosphere seemed to go on for hours and I was absolutely knackered—there was nothing we could do but keep pressing on. The bales outside the barn which we had chucked out were now burning more brightly than the fire inside the barn and the flames were leaping up the wall. I yelled to Doreen to ring the fire brigade and also Roy Muskin, who was one of the villagers who I knew would rush up and help. But she didn't have time to do it and it was literally all down to us to get the blaze under control.

By this time it was dark, and because Jackie's place was the last in the village and on the blind side, no one saw the fire. Anyhow, I think we got the last of the smouldering straw out by around midnight—we had been at it about *11 hours* on the trot. Only the first few hours were total panic, then we knew we could tackle the rest of the fire by damping down the remaining straw. Even the following morning, when I went out to check things, the straw outside was still smouldering, although the fire inside had been well extinguished.

Of course, when it was all over, Kevin and his friend were worried what Jimmy would say when he came home to find his straw all burned, fortunately he was very understanding. I think we could have supplied a complete football match crowd with baked potatoes in their jackets that night!

That was my first real bit of activity on returning to a new life! The boys may have had their worries about Jimmy's return, but Doreen and I had more to worry about. Although I had managed not to get myself burned by the fire, at one stage the flooring upstairs had given way and my leg went through it, and I gashed it on the jagged ends of wood. We knew that I had been lucky not to have fallen through, but I was terrified about what Papworth would say, so I didn't even tell them. Fortunately, my leg didn't become infected and I was able to make light of my injury on my next clinic visit. Mind you, had it become infected, I would have had a right rollocking from Papworth for not reporting it immediately! I was silly not to say anything, but it was early days. Now, if anything goes wrong, I report it immediately; these situations are unavoidable.

Good always comes out of something like that and, on reflection, I was so happy to know that I could get enough oxygen in my lungs to hold my breath and rush about, chucking the burning straw out before I dashed out again. I hadn't been able to hold my breath for *years* and I never thought I would be able to do it again. And to be able to toss 60 lb bales of hay out of an upstairs door to the ground gave me a lot of satisfaction!

One day, Mr English said he was a little concerned that I had not had a biopsy for some time. Although he felt there was no reason to worry he thought I had better come into hospital for that examination, so he made all the arrangements. I decided that, immediately after the biopsy, I would travel to London to sort out the purchase of a small car and the matter of our housing, and then return to Jackie's farm. Mr English, however, didn't like this idea. 'Is Doreen going to travel with you?' I replied in the negative. 'Well, Keith,' he said, 'I'm not keen for you to travel on your own, and even if someone went with you, I'm not keen on you using public transport and hanging about in the bad weather we are now experiencing.' Mr English therefore made sure that, when Sue took me back to Caxton Gibbet, I got on the bus back to the farm, and didn't get the train to London!

Anyhow, back at the farm I said to Doreen; 'Look, love, we've got to get to London. Let's go down tomorrow without saying anything to anybody and keep it nice and quiet.' However, the next day I travelled to London on my own. I can't exactly remember why Doreen didn't

110

come with me. I wish she'd have come with me, because then I wouldn't have landed myself in hot water. Whilst I was away, lo and behold, John Edwards rang the farm and asked to speak to me urgently. He wanted to warn me that the Press could arrive at the farm as another heart transplant operation had just been done at Papworth (on Andrew Barlow). Automatically, Doreen replied: 'Sorry, Mr Edwards—he's up in London.' There was a pause whilst John took this in. 'I thought Mr English said he couldn't go to London,' he answered. Doreen knew she had made a *faux pas*. So I was well and truly caught breaking the rules for the first time. But it was worth it to know that Andrew had undergone his op.

The next day, I was back at Papworth for my clinic. As I was walking down the corridor, I saw Joan Barlow, Andrew's mother, sitting at the end of the corridor, looking for all the world like Rodin's statue, 'The Thinker'. Naturally, I knew Joan from the time when both Andrew and I were being assessed. I crept up to her and said: 'I bet you're feeling happy right now!' She gave a yell, flung her arms around me and we danced round and round in the corridor. All the nurses were very sweet about it. It was such a happy moment for the pair of us. Later on in the day I looked through the window of the 'bubble' to see Andrew, and he looked up and waved at me—naturally, he was still very woozy, and I knew there was plenty of time for conversations later. All that mattered was that Andrew was alive and doing well.

My bi-weekly visits to clinics continued. One day, when I was waiting in the lay-by for Sue to come and collect me, a blue car pulled up opposite me. At first I thought it was Sue, but there were two fellows sitting in it. The car did a wild 'U' turn in the road and pulled up beside me. It turned out to be two chaps from the London *Evening News*. They asked me what I was doing waiting there. I explained my usual routine to them and they expressed amazement that I was hanging about in the damp weather. I said it was quite normal and, soon enough, Sue arrived. She waited whilst the lads took pictures of me pretending to be thumbing a lift, it was all a bit over-exaggerated, but they meant no harm. I told the lads that I was going to London in two days' time to pick up my own car—a real old banger. Sure enough, being good reporters, they asked for the name of the garage and of the friend who was selling me the car and, true to form, they were there to cover the story when I collected it! They wanted me to pose for the usual gimmicky picture—me peering out from under the bonnet. As I was posing away, I rested my hand on the grille when, much to everyone's amusement, the perishing thing fell off! The first picture was therefore of me with my arm through a great rusty hole in the vehicle! It really was a banger! Doreen and I were going to make our way back to Northampton in the car after we had completed the formalities of taxing the car at County Hall. Now, everybody who has had to go through this procedure at County Hall knows the difficulties. It's a very busy place and there is little parking space available. This day was no exception so I parked up the road, leaving Doreen in the car, whilst I whipped into County Hall and performed the necessary tasks with the minimum possible delay. As I came out, Doreen was talking to a traffic warden who waved at me and grinned. I guessed something was up. Sure enough, he had come to give us a ticket for parking in a restricted area. Doreen had explained to him what was going on and he, good as gold, let us off! I must admit that that was the *only* time that I have used my transplant operation as a means of getting out of a tricky situation.

The most pleasurable bit of that trip was still to come—my first visit to St George's. First of all we went down to the basement, where the cardiac department was. The first person we saw was Sister Smith who I was going to see often at clinics. As far as I know, she is still in charge of the Cardiac Unit today. Next I saw Polly, one of the nurses, and she took me to a room full of old familiar faces. Everyone was delighted to see me. It was wonderful shaking hands with them all and listening to how pleased they were about my operation and how much they had all been behind me at the time. I thanked everybody for their support—it was a really happy reunion.

Next stop was Harris Ward, to see Maggie and all the nurses. What a welcome I had. After all the hugs and kisses, questions and answers, Maggie pulled out the largest bottle of vermouth that I have ever seen. (Maggie wouldn't have been Maggie if she hadn't had something up her sleeve!) All the nurses, Doreen and myself and the doctors had a drink to celebrate my homecoming to Harris Ward. Maggie was so generous with her pouring of the vermouth that I had to ask her to go easy, as I thought it might look a bit bad if I were to be breathalised whilst driving up the motorway in the car that I had just bought that day! After a lovely time we had to leave for Northampton, but we knew that we were all going to see more of each other as I would have to attend St George's for clinics on my return to London.

We arrived back at the farm. The following morning I again had to attend a clinic at Papworth and, when I awoke, I heard a bit of a racket going on outside my window. I looked out and, to my amazement, there were newspaper reporters milling about all over the place. The 'no go' area certainly wasn't functioning as all the chaps were up the top end of the drive, inspecting my little car. Of course they had all read about it in the *Evening News*. Jimmy went wild and started talking about the 'invasion of privacy' but I said it wasn't worth the hassle. I advised that he should let them in and give them a coffee, then let them take pictures before I left for Papworth. This is what we did. They photographed me every whichway—with Doreen being helped into the car, me peering through the hoar-frost on the windscreen, and various other poses. Soon it was time for me to go. But, now it happened—the bloody car wouldn't start! The Press, of course, thought it would make a great picture if I was given a bump start down the drive! Well, the drive was very muddy indeed and we hadn't gone more than a few yards when the mud spewing up off the wheels and, not being as fit as Brendan Foster, the first two or three of them started falling by the wayside. The car just wouldn't start! By the time we reached the end of the drive there was only one poor stalwart left pushing! I felt so sorry for him! Then I took pity on him because, all the time I had been taking the mickey out of those reporters and had not turned the key in the ignition! When I saw there was only one chap left I turned it on and the engine burst into life. I waved my hand and thanked him, but I suppose I should really apologise to them all, but I just couldn't resist playing one practical joke!

One photographer even followed me all the way to Papworth, leaning out of the window to see if anything would happen to my car, but nothing did and I had a successful journey to the hospital. There was now more to look forward to, as I had the added pleasure of visiting young Andrew in the 'bubble' after I had finished my clinic. Also Harry Lowe was back there at that time and he promised that when he had his transplant the three of us would have a lovely trip around the west coast of England in his yacht. Alas, it was never to be.

During the course of this clinic, Mr English asked me if I would be prepared to attend a clinical lecture at Addenbrooke's Hospital. He knew that on the day of this lecture I was going to London to see my first Fulham match and that my son-in-law was going to drive me down with Kevin. Of course I agreed, as the lecture was early in the morning. Mr English then suggested that I should stay overnight at Papworth, then Andrew Thorpe and Woggie would drive me to Addenbrooke's on the morning of the lecture. Jimmy could drive over to Addenbrooke's and meet me afterwards and we could then go down to London. This was agreed.

On the appointed day, Woggie, Andrew and I arrived at Addenbrooke's and started making preparations, putting up the screen for the slides, etc. The arrangement was that several doctors from Papworth would present various parts of the lecture according to their departments. I pointed out to Andrew that I was only required to come in at the end and be examined like a prize Hereford bull. 'Can't I come in and listen to the lecture too?' I asked. Andrew said this wouldn't be allowed, but suggested that I could creep into the projection room as one of my old mates from Papworth would be operating the equipment—no one would know I was there. He said he would give me a cue when I was to come forward. So I sat in the projection room and found it all very interesting.

Firstly, Mr Cooper did his bit on the drugs side. He was followed by someone from Pathology and then Andrew had to explain the surgical side. When he came to the part when he showed a picture of me lying on the operating table with my chest cavity wide open, no heart inside, looking like a bit of butcher's meat, Andrew, knowing full well that I was watching, turned to the assembled audience and said: 'Now, gentlemen, we come to the point of no return!' I knew that was for my benefit; it was a good build up. I was very interested to hear the rest of the lecture with all the statistics of transplants world wide. Then it was my turn to go into the hall. I must say that everybody was extremely nice to me. However this was, of course, my first experience of 'an audience' since the operation and I had already become aware that numerous organisations were anxious for me to endorse their products. There were other people too, who, because I was a National Health patient, thought they had the right to extract their pound of medical flesh out of me, as far as my post-operational activities were concerned. I had told Doreen that we would have to be careful what we said and did in order to avoid any arguments over ethics until we knew what was what. So, I was a little wary when I faced this audience of medical people. I think, in retrospect that I may have been a little sharp in answering some questions, particularly when one doctor asked me about smoking. I put the ball firmly back in Mr English's court as I wasn't going to get involved in any argument or endorse anything like that until I knew the score. On the whole, it passed off quite well, but I think I could have handled it better if it had happened today, as I am now so used to speaking to people and I now realise that it is far better to give a true answer and be yourself than to try to answer in the way that is expected of you. Now I think that I am a normal human being who has been lucky enough to be chucked back into life. Before I never thought that I would have much of a life, if one at all.

Afterwards, when we were having coffee, whilst I was waiting for Jimmy, I was far more at ease than I was in the hall—it was far less formal and easier for me to answer questions put to me by the various people who had attended the lecture. Eventually, Jimmy and Kevin arrived and off we went to London where we met Keith, and the four of us arrived at Fulham where we had a really wonderful reception. The teams, both Fulham and West Ham, presented me with a signed ball and there were many jokes about me predicting the score. Well, although I love Fulham, I was a realist and predicted that West Ham would win, 4-2. I wasn't far wrong either! We were treated to lunch by the Mayor of Hammersmith in the stand and Ernie Clay came up to me for a chat and asked if I would do the half time draw, on the pitch, which I did. We had a wonderful time!

After the match, we dropped Keith off and the three of us started back for Northampton. As we were travelling up the M1, I started getting some pains in the left side of my back. These pains started getting worse and worse and, in the end, they were *agony*. When we arrived at the farm, I couldn't even get out of the car and had to be carried out, and, when we got inside, I fell on the floor, writhing about. Everyone was in a state of panic, wondering what was wrong. I thought it was because, having been in a low-slung sports car for the journey, I had been jolted and my back muscle had been pulled as the result but, to make sure, we rang Papworth. The duty surgeon said I had better go to Northampton General straight away (I couldn't make the journey to Papworth in that condition) and said that he would ring them to warn them of my arrival.

We arrived at Northampton General, went to the reception and the next minute I was being examined by a doctor. Everybody was a bit worried because, by then, my body had arched up. I told the doctor (although I knew they hated patients making diagnoses) that I was sure it was a badly pulled muscle, at least that's what it felt like. However, with the drugs I was on, there was a chance that it could have been something else. So there followed X-rays, ECGs, blood tests, etc, and all the results were passed on to Papworth.

The most hilarious part about it was, whilst one of the nurses was wheeling me down a corridor to the X-ray department, a porter said to her: ''Ere, I hear we've got that heart transplant chap in the hospital somewhere—he's collapsed—I hope he's going to make it!' The nurse and I looked at each other and burst out laughing and, luckily, I was able to tell the porter that I did survive and that I had suffered a pulled muscle. They gave me some medicament for this and the next day I had to go to Papworth for further checks, just to be doubly sure.

Between this time and Christmas, Doreen and I made a couple of visits home, to London, to start making arrangements for our return there and also to prepare for our move to another house when we did get back. We had a very quiet Christmas back on the farm. It was probably the most old fashioned Christmas that we had had for a long time—just visiting old friends and taking things very easy. It made me realise how much you miss out at Christmas time when you live in a town. It was yule logs and everything that year.

Soon after Christmas, we returned to London. From now on, our lives were going to be completely different. Up until then we had been sheltered from meeting too many people, and, of course, for the last three years I had been in various intensive care hospital wards and, although I had gone through many *Only When I Laugh* situations, hospital life had been basically very serious. From this moment on, I was to get back to normal life. All I had to do was attend out-patient clinics, where the life-saving aspect was not so predominant. These were at St George's, twice a week, and every time I went there I hopped up to Harris Ward to see all my old friends there, particularly Percy.

For heart transplant patients, there is a way of counting up the ECG recordings and using it as a preliminary means of finding out whether the heart is being rejected or not. On one particular day at one of these clinics, poor old Bill had an absolute fit when he counted my ECG recordings to find that they were only a quarter of what they should have been. He telephoned me at home to ask if I could come in the next day to repeat the test. I went back and fortunately it was the machine which was wrong, not me! This made me realise, however, just how important these clinics were.

Of course I began to meet more and more members of the general public and they all asked questions about my experience. At least when the medical profession asks questions you know there is a good reason for it, but some of the questions I was asked by the public were so wild and woolly it was unbelievable! Many's the time I had a good laugh about them. One lovely comment came from one of the ladies who ran the canteen at St George's. I had just attended a clinic and had found out that another transplant operation had been carried out at Papworth—in fact, it turned out to be Nigel Olney. I was so pleased for him that, when I went to the canteen afterwards for a cup of coffee and a doughnut, I had a huge grin on my face. 'You're looking very chuffed today,' said the lady serving. I pointed to my heart and said: 'Yes, they've done another heart transplant.' 'What!' she exclaimed, 'they're letting you walk about already?' It was marvellous. This was just the sort of misconception which I was going to hear for a long time to come.

The nicest thing to happen in my new life was the addition to our family of our latest grand-daughter, Alex. It was so nice that she was born at St George's—one of the hospitals which had done so much for me. This may seem like slushy sentiment to you, but the world's a better place for a bit of sentiment—there is far too much callousness about. Everyone in St George's was over the moon about Alex's birth, as were Wendy and Dominic, her parents, and young Alex was certainly welcomed into the world with a lot of Press ballyhoo! But it was done in such a lovely way.

After Nigel Olney had had his heart transplant operation, they performed one on Ewan McPhee, but there is a story about him which we laughed about for months afterwards. Going back to the time when I was in Papworth and was about to attend the lecture at Addenbrooke's, Mr English, with a rather old fashioned look, asked me if I had spoken to Mr McPhee yet. I twigged right away that Euan was up for an assessment, so I said that I certainly would have a word with him. It was my policy, once a heart transplant operation was to go ahead, to try to reassure the patient by telling him about my own experiences. So I managed to get Euan out of the ward and started talking to him about transplants in general. I asked him: 'Has Mr English said "yes" yet?' He looked at me blankly. 'Crikey,' I thought, 'he doesn't have a clue what I'm talking about, he doesn't *know*. I'd better back off—I must have got the wrong end of the stick from Mr English!' So, I quickly changed the subject and walked away, hoping that Euan would not think me some kind of nut case. However, the next morning he came to my room and said he had just twigged that he was at Papworth for a possible transplant—he hadn't realised this before. However, he didn't like the idea and wanted some time to go away and think about it. Mr English agreed to this and said that, if Euan's condition deteriorated, he could come back to Papworth for his operation. So, it was a pleasant surprise to learn that he had in fact had his transplant.

Soon after that there were a couple more operations—on John Power and Paul Coffey—and I was over the moon about all these patients getting new hearts. It was wonderful. A ball had started rolling, and I hoped this would go on for evermore. Unfortunately, one person who wasn't getting his transplant was poor old Harry. This was at the back of my mind all the time—why was he being passed over? It was this situation that made me think about predestination. Is your path in life mapped out? Of course, every time I went to a clinic in Papworth there were more and more transplantees with their families and more people waiting for assessment with their families and it was beginning to feel like a club. Also in London, at my twice-weekly clinics, I was always bumping into old friends as well.

By now, Bill Ginks had marked Percy's card and informed him that it was time they started considering him for a transplant but it was, as usual, all a matter of whether he could stand the operation. Although you might not have known that Percy was ill to look at him, both he and his sons had told me of occasions when he had collapsed on the floor, but he never talked to others about it.

About two or three months after I had returned to London I got severe chest pains all of a sudden. I rang St George's and they asked me to come in. I don't know why, but we packed some clothing. Doreen and I must have had a premonition because the pains were quite bad. Sure enough, it was back to my old bed in Harris Ward, where pneumonia was diagnosed.

Now infection is the fear of any transplantee. Most people think that *rejection* is our big dread, but *infection* is a bigger cause for concern, particularly a chest infection which can run riot. They were very concerned at St George's and, having seen a couple of specialists, I found myself transferred to Papworth Hospital. The first time I had journeyed to Papworth it had been by train and kitchen van; this time it was very different, I had an ambulance, a police escort and the whole works! Funnily enough, one of the policemen on escort duty was a drinking friend of mine from my local, *The Fox and Hounds*. I didn't even recognise him as I was rushed so quickly to the ambulance on the stretcher that I just didn't notice him.

On arrival at Papworth, the team were waiting for me. There were lots of checks and tests and Mr English looked very concerned. He was in consultation with the chest specialist from Addenbrooke's all the time and the following day I had further tests which involved putting an optic tube down into my lungs. Actually, they had attempted this test when I arrived, but I had vomited when the tube went down my throat so the doctor quickly withdrew it and I had to have a further bronchoscopy the following day under full theatre conditions. I didn't mind, but I *was* upset when Mr English criticised me about being a bit lackadaisical in reporting my present condition. In retrospect I knew that he had told me off because he was concerned and worried about me. Anyhow, they managed to get on top of the pneumonia and I recovered. I was very pleased about this, as it was the first time after suffering a secondary illness that I had been able to shrug it off. Before I left for London, Mr English again tried to tell me off and he stressed the urgency of reporting any minor illness. He wasn't really much good at telling people off and I had a little grin to myself on the way home, but his intentions were, as usual, for the best. He could have punched me on the nose and I would have forgiven him straight away.

Human nature being what it is, with people wanting to be superior to their fellows, I now ran into the 'one-upmanship brigade' (as far as surgical operations were concerned). I met many people who *swore* they had had eight by-passes or ten valve replacements all in one go—the type of extraordinary operation which would have made Mr English's eyes stand out on stalks! The best example of this occurred, in *The Fox and Hounds*. I was standing in there one day, talking to a friend of mine, when I felt a little tug at my sleeve. I turned and found a small woman standing beside me. 'You're 'im, ain't yer?' she said. 'Well, yes,' I replied, knowing what she meant. She immediately launched into a long tale about how her husband had had the first wonder heart operation and how the surgeons were astounded about how much he could stand and so I asked, after stating how pleased I was, 'How is your husband now?' 'Oh,' she said brightly, 'he's dead!' My friend, Ginger, and I managed to keep straight faces, but that is now Ginger's favourite heart joke!

I next heard of an unfortunate incident concerning Nigel Olney. It was largely due to misguidedness on the part of the people who loved him as they tried to do their best for him. It was decided that there would be a new discharge system at Papworth. Instead of the patient spending his full ten-week recovery time at Papworth, at the end of eight weeks and following a biopsy with satisfactory results, the patient would be returned to his local hospital to get used to receiving more visitors and to get back more easily to the routine of everyday living. At the end of a fortnight, he had to return to Papworth for a final biopsy and then be released home.

Arrangements were made for Nigel to go to his local hospital in London and they, being extra wary of their patient and trying to do the very best for him, slapped him straight back into a Barrier Room and visitors were frowned upon except his nearest and dearest, and I had great difficulty in getting to see him myself. In desperation, I turned to one of the nurses and said: 'Look, love, there's nothing going on in that room that I ain't seen before.' They let me in. However, Nigel told me that he was worried that something had gone wrong because he had been put back in a Barrier Room and he didn't realise that they were only giving him tender loving care and attention in order to safeguard him from something going wrong. Luckily, Andrew Thorpe was visiting London at the time and he called in to see Nigel. Andrew reported back to TE but, by the time he was told the story, the fortnight was up and it was back to Papworth for Nigel. The same thing happened to John Power when he went back to his local hospital in Manchester, so, after that, all local hospitals were told that intense barrier nursing wasn't necessary. It just shows you that heart transplants were a rare breed of patient and that the nursing staff had to learn how to handle them. You can't blame them for wanting to do the best for their patients.

We had now been in our new house in Battersea for a couple of months and I had been doing various jobs to make it 'home'. I had broken up some old concrete in the garden and roughly set it out how we wanted it. We had also sown some grass seed and had generally done up the garden. We were quite pleased with the house and, with a few additions to our old furniture, things became very comfortable.

Many charitable institutions now approached me with a view to my helping their fund-raising activities by making personal appearances. At first they felt it was a bit of an imposition to ask me to give up my time to do this sort of thing, but *I* felt all along that I had been incredibly lucky and wanted to help others. How could I possible have refused these requests? This will always be my attitude. However, when it came to heart transplants, I soon found that I really had to watch myself and take care of how I spoke to people who were up for assessment for the operation. This came about because of Paul Coffey.

I first met Paul about three weeks after he had his first heart attack and, quite naturally, being young with a pregnant wife, he was a bit down in the dumps. He asked about the operation and I told him the absolute truth. I said: 'Paul, it's absolutely marvellous! I had no pain whatsoever—not one iota and I couldn't cough up any sputum when they asked me, my lungs were in such good nick. It was a clear straight run for me.' Well, about four weeks later, Paul had his transplant, remembering what I had said all the time. However, following the operation his chest did give him some pain. This is quite natural when you consider the method of opening the chest but some patients were obviously going to get a little bit bruised and sore while others felt nothing at all. I only told him of my own experiences. Poor Paul, lying in quite a bit of pain, waved his fist in the air and said to his young wife: 'Wait till I get my hands on that bloody Keith Castle—telling me there was no pain indeed—I'll really give him what for!' But he was really happy to be fit and alive and he knew really that you have to expect that sort of pain when your muscles have been pulled round quite a bit. Actually, I think Paul is probably the fittest of us all, I don't remember him having any setbacks at all. I hope he keeps it up, especially as at the time of writing this, Sue is expecting another babe. In fact, Paul will be the only heart transplant patient to become a father after his operation. I always said Coffey would do anything to get into the headlines—and there you are! What could be a better endorsement for the transplant programme than a nice young couple behaving like any other young parents?

It was soon time for the annual Papworth fête and, behind the scenes, all those dedicated staff were working hard. Everyone put themselves out to make it a most enjoyable day and, of course, raise a bit of cash. Alma, who first came to Papworth as a TB patient was also about to retire. (For those of you who don't know the history of the hospital, Papworth was originally a TB hospital in this resettlement village. A lot of the staff, including nurses, were in fact ex-TB patients.) When we heard about Alma's retirement, we decided that we would have a quick whip-round and buy her a silver salver, engraved with all the names of the heart transplant patients to date.

Alma knew nothing of our plans and, during the fête, we called her over. Andrew Patterson, who was the latest recipient of a new heart, and who had been a very sick young man indeed and was still not out of the woods, had received permission from TE to come outside to present the salver to her. He was sitting in a wheelchair, still with his mask on, and the rest of us gathered round to watch the little ceremony. Alma was overwhelmed and told me later that she would never forget this experience. I am very glad to say that Andrew made an excellent recovery and in fact he and Paul Coffey went to represent Papworth Hospital at the Transplant Olympic Games held in Greece.

It was a lovely day for all of us. We put Paul in the stocks and pelted him with wet sponges, and indulged in all the usual fête activities. True to form, it even rained, but it didn't dampen our spirits. As a matter of fact, there was a nice little dance in the grounds of Papworth Hospital afterwards which was enjoyed by all. This was the first fête at Papworth (1980) which I attended after my operation and I am pleased to say that I have now been to four in total—one every year. Since then, fêtes and charity functions have become part of my life and I spend a lot of time travelling up and down the country to attend them.

Soon after this fête at Papworth, I had a most enjoyable trip to Harefield Hospital to see Derek Morris before he was let out into the world. This was a real time for celebration for Harefield were sending their first heart transplant patient home. To me it was a wonderful sign that at last heart transplants were becoming an accepted medical procedure. I am pleased to say that this was the start of an association which I have kept up with Harefield. The marvellous thing about attending these hospital functions is that I am seeing more and more new people who have gone through the operation successfully or waiting hopefully for the chance of a transplant. It has been a pipe-dream of mine that one day all the transplant patients would get together—not for a big binge or anything like that—but just so we could meet each other and catch up on old friendships. However, geographically, we are well spread out. Anyway, if we don't get together soon, there will be far too many of us to find a meeting place, when you think of the number of successful operations which have taken place and the number of transplants to come.

June of that year was very eventful for me. St George's, Hyde Park, was finally about to close as the move over to Tooting neared completion. During the week of my last visit to the clinic at Hyde Park, Doreen and I were to make a long journey up north, where we were to attend a function in York and another one in Harrogate—we also thought we would look in on Andrew Barlow in Leeds at the same time—so St George's arranged to keep a couple of departments open for me so that I could attend a clinic on my return.

From York, we drove to Leeds and spent the evening with the Barlows and had a most enjoyable time. Naturally, they wanted us to stay overnight, but we had to press on to Harrogate and the cycle show. Now, just before this show, to my complete and utter surprise, I had been elected 'Cyclist of the Year'. Believe it or not, in second place was Jimmy Carter and in third place—the Pope! It tickled me to find myself in front of these eminent people and I had visions of Jimmy Carter riding knee deep in peanuts and The Holy Father, his robes tucked up à la Gandhi, frantically cycling around the Vatican! Anyway we had a wonderful time at the cycle show and enjoyed meeting the executives of this industry. You certainly don't expect to see so many trim figures on a Board of Directors, but these executives are still keen cyclists, and they have a very athletic approach to their business!

We left Harrogate on the Thursday morning and belted down the motorway because I had arranged to get back to Hyde Park Corner for my clinic by mid-day. This was to be my last one at that venue. I felt somehow humbled by the fact that this great hospital, closing now after so many years of dedicated service, had kept open three departments just for me to have these final tests—ECG, haemotology and X-ray. I must say I was tired and hot when I arrived at the hospital that lunchtime, and it was like walking through a mausoleum. Our footsteps echoed in the corridors which I had known to bustle with activity. Several of the nurses were having a little sentimental weep and we never did do my tests, but just sat around drinking tea and reminiscing. We took photographs of each other and I told everyone how honoured I felt to be the very last patient in this great hospital which, to many including myself, is the finest heart hospital in the world. I know there are equally good training hospitals in London such as Bart's, Guy's and St Thomas's, but there can be only one 'best' and I think it is St George's. I shall certainly have egg on my face, having said this, when I go to Bart's hospital with Dave Haggar, another Papworth 'transplantee' but originally a Bart's patient. Dr Bexton will send me away with a flea in my ear, I'll bet! But the truth will be out—for me St George's is *the best*.

9

Where did those two years go?

The realisation slowly dawned on Doreen and me that it was almost a year since I had had my transplant—time had flown by and we had had a marvellous time with everyone being so kind. The newspapers began to telephone me about my forthcoming celebration. It was amazing to me that ordinary people living in an ordinary little house in Battersea could get so much attention from the media—on one day, the reporters were literally queuing up outside for an interview! Both television companies came to do stories, too, and, whilst one did an interview with me in the back garden, the other one was in our front room awaiting its turn. There were newspaper reporters and photographers all over the place, in the house, out in the front street—it was just like our first Press conference at Papworth all over again. However, it was a very important occasion, it was my first 'MOT' as it were.

It was at Papworth that these celebrations were nicest. The chef had baked me a cake—I am sure he must have cleared the Cambridge Area Health Authority out of fruit and currants, because it was the biggest cake I had ever seen. This was brought to me after I had the usual ECG and angiogram tests and all was found to be in order. The chef and I took ages to cut up part of the cake, which soon disappeared. I must say the greediest so and so's of the lot were the surgeons—they kept coming back for second and third helpings and, being handy with the scalpel, they could cut themselves pieces of cake in no time at all! This was undoubtedly a landmark for Papworth Hospital—the first anniversary of their first heart transplant patient. I was pleased for the hospital, the staff and, of course, for myself! What a success my op had proved to be.

As far as my tests were concerned, I was not too worried about the biopsy report because there had been no problems so far and no signs of rejection, but I was far more interested in the reports about my arteries and wanted to know how I was faring regarding cholesterol. Mr Cory-Pearce, who was running the research unit, came to congratulate me on my first year and my good results. The only thing wrong was that one little artery was blocked up, however, this was fairly unimportant. He did ask me to eat less cholesterol and then we would see if we could correct things by the next anniversary.

Mr English also expressed pleasure at my progress and, although he was still waiting for the secondary results of the biopsy, he said I could go home, the primary results being OK. I had already dropped Doreen off to stay with one of the ladies in the village and, as it was a bit late, I said I would hang on until the morning.

I waited about the hospital that night and stopped to talk to Mavis Britain. Her son, Richard, was at that time very poorly indeed. (I know that Mavis and her husband, Tony, don't mind me talking frankly about this.) I think Tony had accepted the inevitability of Richard's illness, but Mavis was waiting to see Mr Cory-Pearce who was going to give her the full details of the situation. What could I say to Mavis? I remember mumbling to her, trying to show my sympathy. I asked why, at 53 years of age, everything had gone so well for me, and yet Richard, who was only 16, seemed to have had no luck at all. Mavis was so wonderful and generous in her response. She told me she would never begrudge me my luck and that she was delighted that everything had worked out the way it had for me. (Mavis's words were to be repeated by many of the next of kin of those patients who did not make it and I marvel that they have all had these wonderful sentiments at a time when it must have been very difficult for them to understand why things had gone so wrong for their own loved ones.)

It was getting quite late and Mavis had to get back to Huntingdon. I asked one of the nurses, Carol, if it would be all right for me to drive her back there after she had seen Mr Cory-Pearce. I assured them that I would take things easily (I had just had an angiogram) and a patient said he would accompany me. The duty surgeon agreed and Carol added that, officially, I was not a patient at Papworth and, as far as she was concerned, TE had discharged me at 7 o'clock that evening.

So, after Mavis had seen Mr Cory-Pearce, I drove her back to Huntingdon with the other patient as company. After we left Mavis at her hotel, we stopped at a takeaway place and took back a little Chinese meal for the night staff, so I spent the evening of my first 'MOT' enjoying my second Chinese meal with the staff of Papworth Hospital.

Soon it was back to what was fast becoming a way of life for Doreen and me—fêtes and functions followed thick and fast, including one function which I was looking forward to very much. Mr English had been elected as one of the 'Men of the Year' and there was to be a large reception at The Savoy. TE had said he was too busy to go to collect his award but, knowing him and the fact that he always shunned publicity, this was no surprise to me. You can imagine how proud I was when he asked me if I would like to go and collect the award on his behalf. Who better to do this than one of his patients? Naturally, I was thrilled. I felt so proud, sitting at this big table with all the other 'Men of the Year' and it was nice to know that people were now taking a great interest in

Right Here I am receiving a cheque for £3,953.10 for Papworth from the Lord Mayor of Norwich on behalf of the taxi drivers of Norwich *(Eastern Daily Press)*.

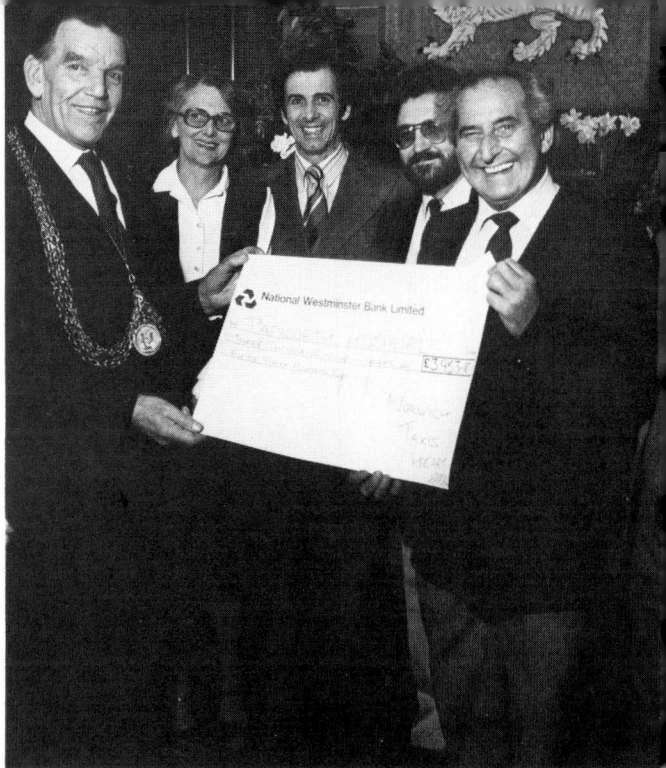

Below With Keith and Doreen in Battersea *(George Konig, Syndication International Ltd)*.

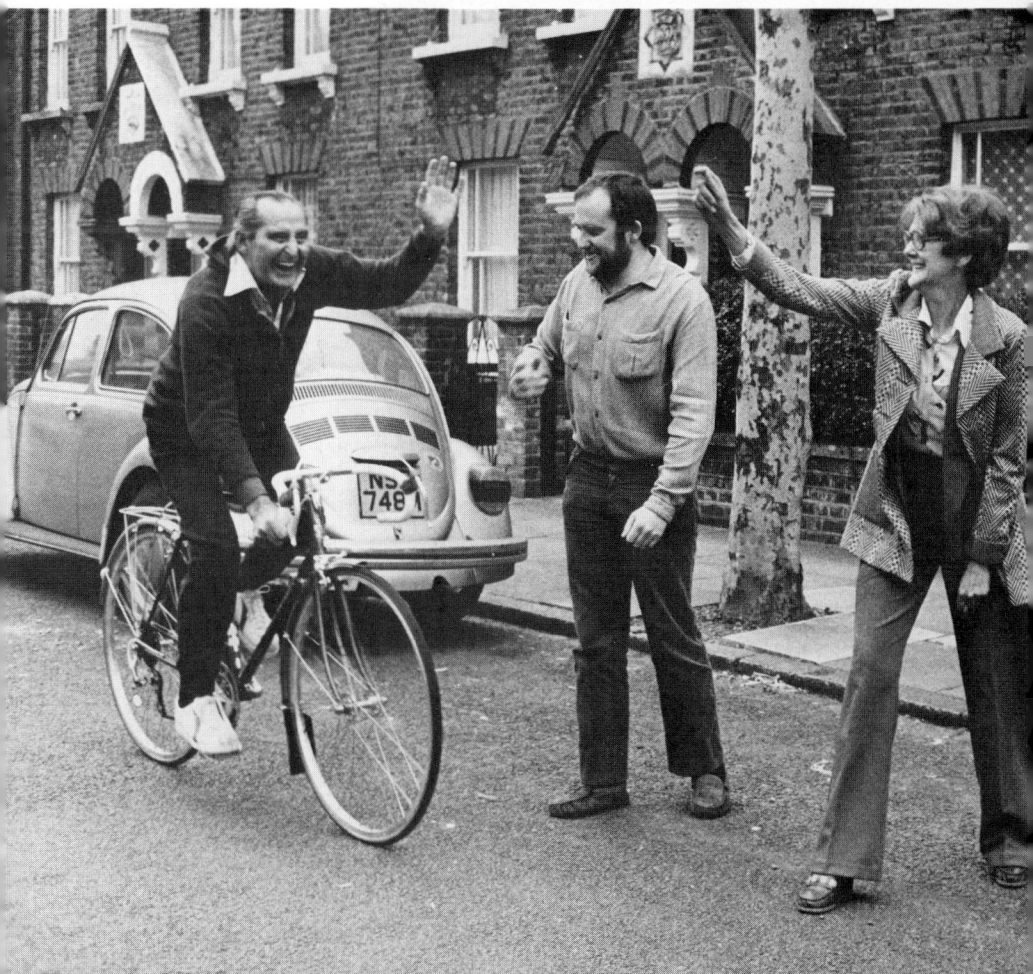

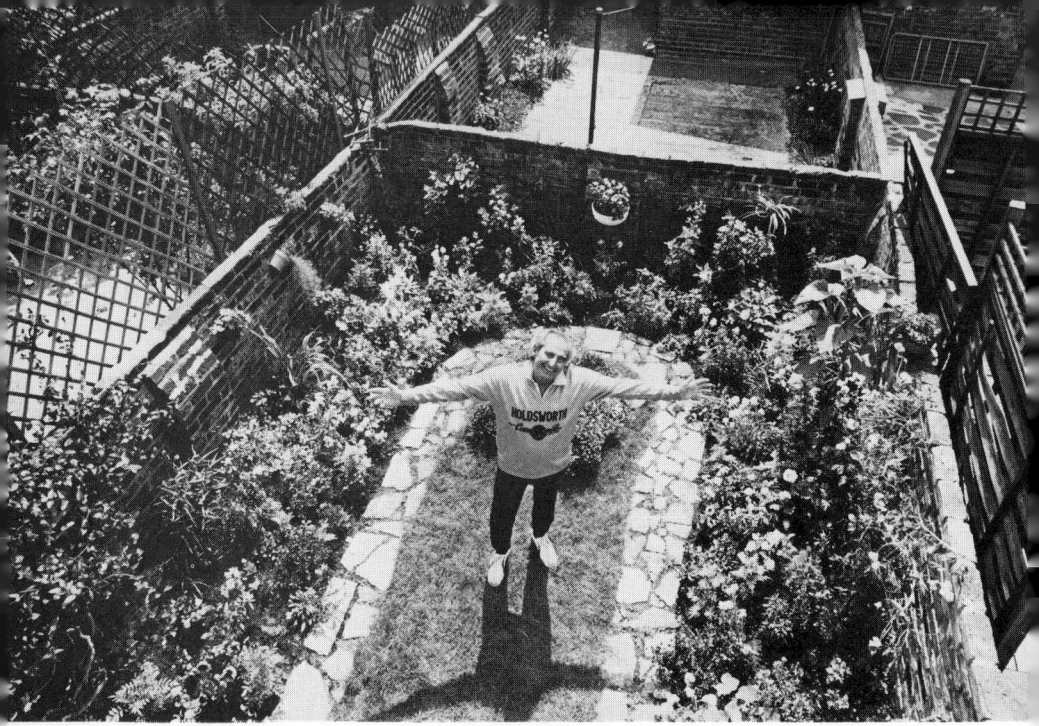

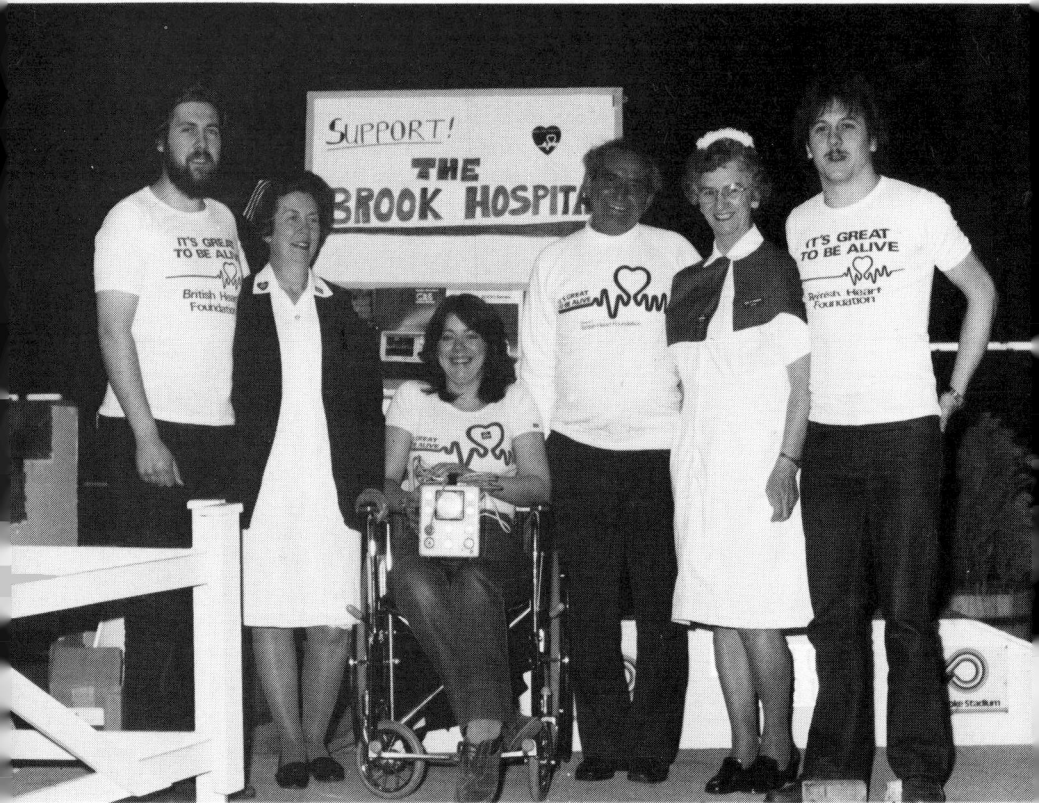

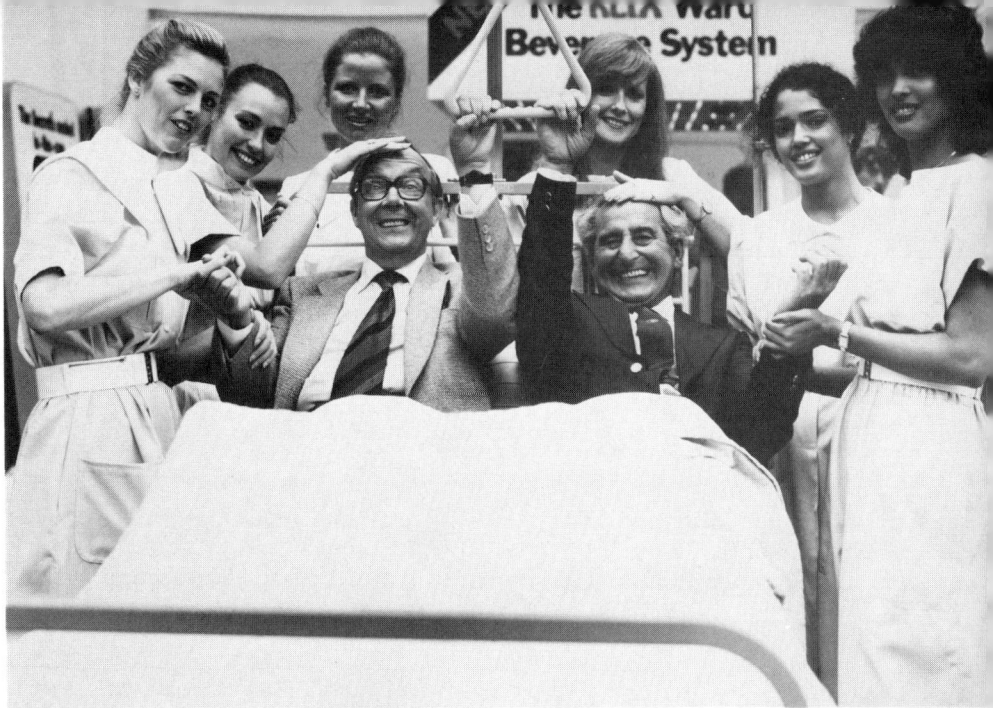

Above left My garden in Battersea.

Left Raising money for the Brook Hospital at Crayford Greyhound Stadium. (The Brook Hospital has had one man and one woman heart transplant patient at Papworth—both operations were successful!)

Above In bed with Eric Morecambe! (The Medical Exhibition, Olympia, 1982) *(Pic Photos)*.

Right Practising for the big race! *(BBC copyright)*.

Overleaf A satisfied customer with a life assurance policy *(Smith & Pinching Ltd, Norwich)*.

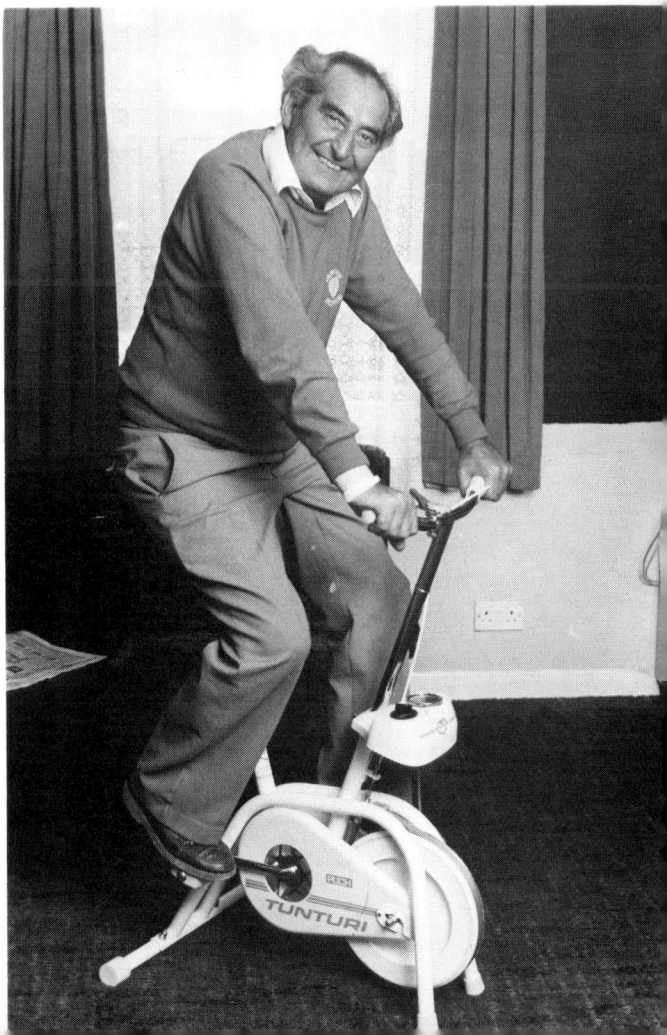

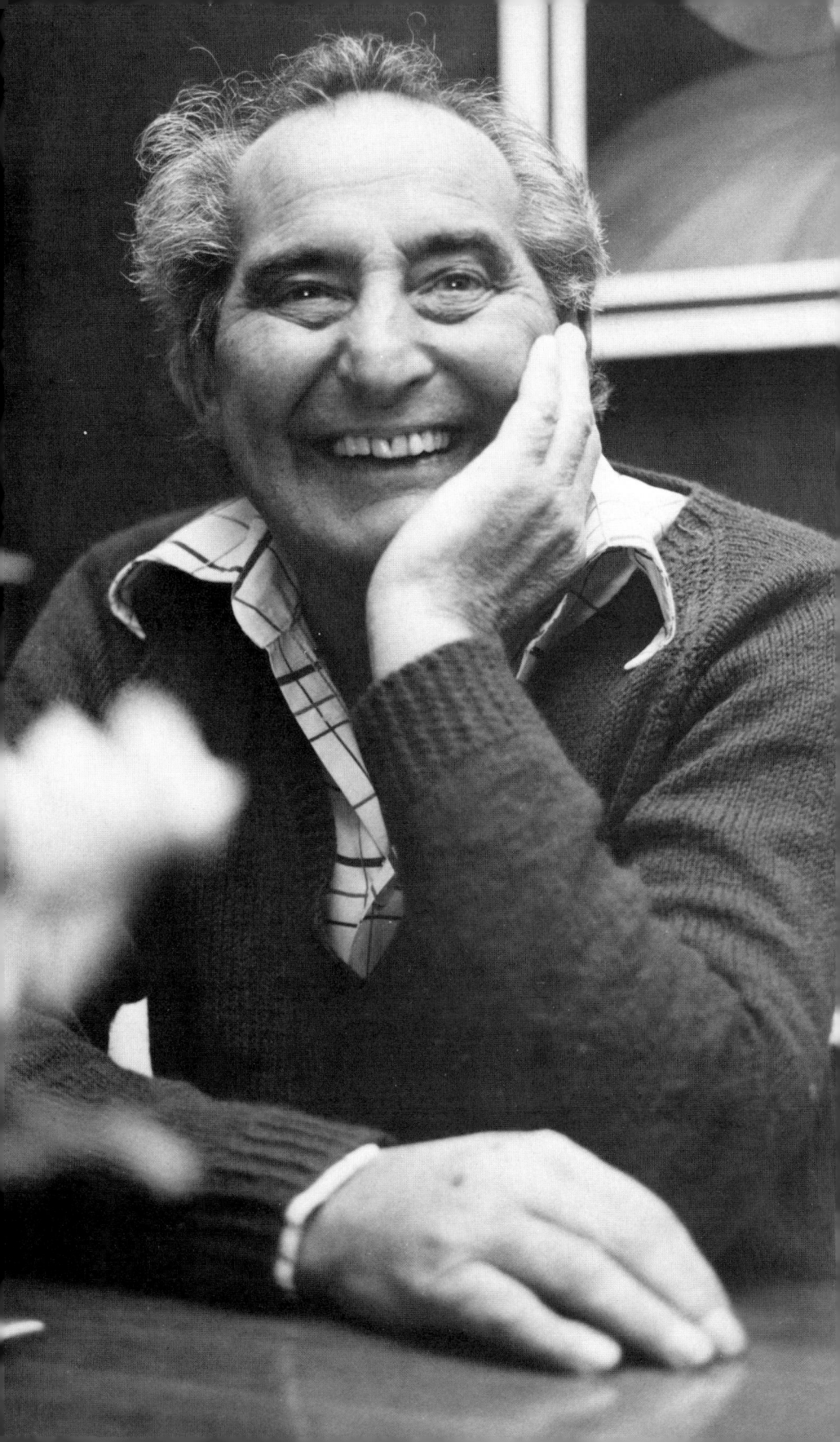

TE's work—so many of them came over to talk to me about him.

Shortly after this I was asked to address a Life Insurance Convention at Wembley. I had to go on the platform and be 'interviewed' by various life insurance agents. During the course of the interview, I threw down a challenge to the agents who dealt with life insurance for heart transplant patients. I wasn't particularly looking for cover for myself as I already had a couple of policies. Following the convention, I was very pleased to hear that I had been awarded a 10-year endowment policy. This was very good news for all heart transplant patients—hard and realistic businessmen were at last prepared to accept us as normal people and offer us insurance cover. We have no difficulty in obtaining car insurance, but I'm afraid I can't say the same thing about driving licences. I really would like to see the rules changed here. I must have been one of the last people to have the old red driving licence, and, when it became time for me to apply for one of the new 'life' licences I was ill, and so declared, as requested on my application form, that I suffered from heart problems.

Now, I must give the Licencing Authority their fair due—they did give me every opportunity to prove that I was capable of driving a car, but it dragged on for 12 months and eventually, I managed to convince them and they gave me a 3-year licence, but that dated from the termination of the old one, so I had already lost a year whilst I proved my point, and I therefore only had two years of that licence to go. When it was time for me to renew this document, quite naturally I thought I would now get a life-long one, but again they only gave me one for 3 years. This is their current practice regarding heart transplantees. I can see that this is really a bureaucratic decision, but, if we are capable of driving a car for 3 years, why can't we drive one for a lifetime? One day things may change.

Anyhow, I felt I was well on the road back to the 'normal' world—I had a driving licence, my car was insured and also my life. But, just before Christmas, bang! No, not a car smash, but I did end up in hospital again—with pneumonia! There was no need for me to go up to Papworth and St George's at Tooting treated me. I had never before had the type of treatment they gave me. I had to wear an oxygen mask and breathe in some type of fine dust which went right into my lungs. I had been examined by Dr Mark Dancey many times and, since the op, had often chatted with him whilst I was an out-patient, but it had been a long time since he had given me a physical examination and this he had to do, because of my pneumonia. During the course of his examination, he grasped my ankles and fell about laughing. 'Keith,' he laughed, 'I just can't get over your skinny ankles!' The realisation of what he had said hit me because the last time he had given me a medical, my legs and ankles had been about ten times their normal size, swollen with liquids

129

and toxins, and now here he was, laughing at my lady-like ankles!

After an operation like a heart transplant, the most obvious benefit is being able to breathe easily and, after a while, you become aware of the other benefits and, when someone who examined you before the operation then remarks on them, you have complete confirmation of the transformation. So, Dr Dancey's comments really pleased me.

I did not have to stay long in St George's on that occasion. Dr Redwood felt that I would be better off at home, now that they had got the pneumonia under control, and I needed no second bidding. This was about the week before Christmas and I recovered quickly.

This Christmas (1980) was similar to last year's—we visited St George's and St James's to see our old friends, particularly Maggie. Whilst visiting St George's, I sought out Professor Pilkington to say a big 'thank you' for all he had done for me. When I did find him, he was in the middle of his rounds, with all the usual retinue following him. He broke off from this when he saw me and we all had a nice little chat. However, I noticed that the old Prof still did his usual trick of putting his hand round my shoulder and slipping his thumb on to my Venus point! But all was well. In fact, having written about 1980 there seemed to have been little in the way of medical goings on—just fêtes, functions and events of that sort! My regular clinics were as much out of academic interest as medical necessity and, week after week, I was pronounced fit.

I attended clinics regularly at Tooting under Dr Redwood and it was here that I noticed a little routine emerge. I used to go into a room beside the clinic, strip to the waist and pull my trousers up to my knees so that my legs could be examined. Dr Redwood would then bring a young doctor in and would casually say to him; 'Oh, just examine that patient—I won't be a couple of minutes.' He would then pop out and the young doctor would start examining me. On seeing the scar down my chest he would know that I had had heart surgery. He would start to ask the usual questions: 'How are you?' 'Oh, fine,' I would answer. 'Well, why are you here?' 'Oh, it's just my clinic attendance.' The doctor in question would look at my notes and then look puzzled as he couldn't find anything wrong with me. Then he would listen to my chest and, just as he was starting to quiz me again, Dr Redwood would come in and say: 'Oh, didn't I tell you? Mr Castle is one of our heart transplant patients.' Just as though there were dozens of us! I was the only one when he started this game! I also noticed that he seemed to play this trick with great enjoyment on young American doctors and I swear the good doctor used to bend down and listen at the keyhole for his 'cue' to make his entrance, looking the picture of innocence! I know I shouldn't accuse my consultants of listening at keyholes and I shall probably get well and truly told off when Dr Redwood reads this, but I did feel it happened like that! I suppose this is the moment to state that I did feel that clinics were fun to go to because I was exceptionally lucky as all my doctors had a keen sense of humour.

During that first year, apart from the pneumonia incident, nothing untoward happened and the clinics became routine. The doctors looked in case little things went wrong. In fact I had a bit of trouble from the side effects of the steroids I was taking and, as I said earlier, I had a lot of painful ulcers in my mouth, but gradually, over a period of six months or so they cleared up but then I started to get ulcers on my legs or arms if I cut or nicked myself. These would take a long time to heal. However, they were all minor things and, when it came to the actual crunch of worrying about my heart, there were no problems and so clinics were a light-hearted affair for me.

The first quarter of 1981 passed much as before but Easter and the following month contained many highlights for me. One day, when a reporter was interviewing me at home, she asked Doreen if she had any ambition. 'Yes,' she replied, 'I'd love to have a chat with Emmanuel Vitrai, the world's longest heart transplant survivor.' Doreen, knowing that Emanuel was French, assumed that he lived in Bologne which was only an inch away from London on the map and didn't realise that he actually lived in Marseilles which was about 1,000 miles away! Anyway, this reporter said she would have a word with her Editor as this would make a good story for the paper. Within a week the whole thing was buttoned up, so we found ourselves with Jean, the journalist and Karl, the photographer in Marseilles!

No one can go to Marseilles without a visit to the famous fish restaurants and we had a lovely meal with the newspaper folk on the first night. The Paris branch manager of the paper flew down to act as an interpreter so, the following day, I was all set for my meeting with Emmanuel. As I waited on the sunny balcony I smoked a quick cigarette. Suddenly, I saw Peter, our 'interpreter' and Emmanuel arrive so I quickly flicked the rest of my cigarette over the side. (Later on I found out that Emmanuel, who was also a smoker, had seen me get rid of my fag so he flicked his away too! Neither of us wanted to take a chance of upsetting each other!)

We began being interviewed by Jean with Karl snapping photographs all the while. However, poor old Peter had a problem on his hands. He wasn't just translating from English to French, he was trying to translate *Cockney* English into *Marseilles* French! Now, Marseilles French is the equivalent to our 'scouse' and, with his impeccable accent in both languages, he did have a bit of a job on! Well, Emmanuel and I had a marvellous time, asking each other questions and comparing notes. He wanted us to stay in Marseilles that night so that he could show us how *Frenchmen* enjoyed a night out, but the arrangements were for us to spend the evening in Paris. It was a wonderful trip organised by the newspaper and we had a lovely time, thoroughly enjoying ourselves and the treats which were laid on for us.

When we returned home, I was sitting one day thinking of Percy. I hadn't heard from him for a while so I decided to telephone. One of his sons answered and I said: 'Is the old reprobate in?' 'No,' was the reply 'haven't you heard? He's in hospital.' 'Good God!' I said, 'what on earth has happened?' 'He's had his transplant! The operation was a few days ago, I'm so sorry, I thought you knew.' Well, it transpired that Grace, his wife, had naturally gone with him to Papworth and everyone thought that I had been told. I immediately 'phoned Percy at Papworth, congratulated him and told him that I would visit him soon. When I eventually did get to see him, Percy being Percy, couldn't help but rub salt into my wounds! He really took the mickey about me not 'phoning before and said: 'Well, if you want to be stand-offish,' etc, etc. We had a laugh about the mix up and I was delighted to say that his op was a success. I was going to see a lot of Percy in the days to come.

The next big event in our lives was the meeting that Doreen and I at last had with Mr and Mrs Prestt. Ever since our visit to York we had been arranging to meet them. We were naturally very nervous, wondering how the Prestts would feel when they met me.

Well, it was a wonderful experience. There was just Ian and Jennifer and their daughter, Julie, to meet us and, far from having a stilted conversation, we even managed to talk about the clinical aspects of the operation. I knew that Doreen was completely at home when she started scrounging flowers from Jennifer! She is the world's greatest addict as far as flower arranging is concerned and would have to be at her ease to scrounge from someone she had never met before! It was a day that I wouldn't have missed for all the world. (Incidentally Emmanual Vitrai has a fortnight's holiday every year with his donor's family.)

In quick succession after that followed the Doctor of the Year Awards, once again at The Savoy. Now, at that time, the BBC were doing a documentary about me—not about the transplant operation, but about how different people react to having been thrust into the headlines. I was to be in one programme of a 6-part series. The BBC were at The Savoy filming the photographers filming me—like a film within a film if you know what I mean.

Doreen and I were really looking forward to it because we were to meet a very gracious lady—Princess Alexandra. Now naturally, Pat Houlahan, the BBC producer, wanted to cover our actual meeting with the Princess—so, when we were presented to her in the foyer, the cameras were all rolling. We then all went into the dining room for the meal. After this was over an incident occurred which I will not forget in a hurry. It shows the graciousness of the young Princess in making ordinary people at their ease. On leaving, Princess Alexandra and her husband, The Hon Angus Olgivy, came over to our table and she stopped to chat to Doreen. Well, of course, this gesture made Doreen's day. I think her mouth is still open about this! You should have seen Pat's face, too, as she had just packed up her camera crew and sent them home when this happened. What a shame, it would have been an excellent bit for her programme! I don't think Doreen's feet touched the ground for the next week—but doesn't it just go to show how marvellous our Royalty are!

Immediately after this we went to my mate Jock's fête at Kings Lynn. Jock Brand had been a heart by-pass patient at Papworth and was trying to raise money for the hospital by organising a fête, which has now developed into an annual event. This year, the particular attraction was Eddie Kidd, the stunt rider, who had made the very generous gesture of offering to appear free of charge. The stunt was—and only Jock could have thought of this—that seven heart transplant patients would lie down and young Eddie would jump over us on his motorcycle.

Unfortunately, due to some error, someone else had booked Eddie Kidd and he was due to perform in a field on the other side of the town. Now, if people had gone there to watch the Eddie Kidd Circus they would have had to pay a certain amount of money for that show whereas they could come to Jock's show, an all-day function at a cheaper rate, and see Eddie Kidd for no extra charge. Quite naturally, this is what they did.

Throughout that day it poured with rain and the field allocated to Eddie's Circus was absolutely waterlogged. In the end he came over to our field, which was not nearly as bad, and did his stunt of riding over the seven of us. Theoretically, he had committed financial suicide because of this whole venture, but I am glad to say that, having made such a grand and spontaneous gesture in performing free, he then had his reward. His unselfish act had attracted a lot of attention from the Press and, the next day, the Council allowed him to move his circus to Jock's field so I do hope he recuperated all his losses of the previous day. Mind you, there were a lot of people who were concerned about us seven patients, just in case anything went wrong. Now, poor Mr Engish was in a bit of a cleft stick. Had it been left to him, I don't think that he would have asked us not to go through with it, but other people put pressure on him. Anyway, I said to Mr English before we started: 'Look, Mr English, I would never let anyone treat me as a red-nosed clown. We are not freaks at a side-show to be stared at, but this fête means a family day out—its kids and slides and roundabouts and swings—and in this sort of environment we can afford to let our hair down a bit more than usual.'

Although Mr English appreciated my view of things, he did come to

133

the fête with a letter in his pocket which asked us not to take part but, after chatting to us over lunch and hearing our views, he didn't produce it. Eddie Kidd's manager assured us that there was no danger and that in fact Eddie could travel a good three times further than was requested on this occasion, but they did some dummy runs to find out when he should open his throttle and, of course, the stunt went off brilliantly. All's well that ends well. I think we all knew by then what sort of functions we could attend with impunity, and for my part, I feel so lucky about my circumstances that I will always attend charitable fêtes and family days out if my help is needed.

However, there is the obvious danger of heart transplant patients being exploited and I did in fact telephone Mr Edwards about a certain offer I had received from a television company. They wanted me to appear in a programme which I felt could have turned into a ribald form of entertainment which was not the image we wanted to portray about Papworth. I decided in the end to pull out of this particular one.

After Jock's fête, Doreen and I had our first holiday. Our local pub, *The Fox and Hounds*, had arranged for us to go to Majorca. (Apparently, if someone organises a block booking, then the party gets two extra seats free.) This year, the two free seats were given to us. So we were off to Majorca with all our friends! Doreen, by now, had overcome her fear of flying, following our trip to see Emmanuel, so this time she felt better and more relaxed about it. We had a wonderful time but, would you believe it, when we went shopping one day someone recognised me and, for about a quarter of a mile uphill on our way back, this berk actually walked backwards, staring at me all the while. I just couldn't understand it. Why didn't he come and talk to me or something? To stare only, walking backwards, was very strange behaviour. I am recognised quite often in the street and people are usually very kind and shake my hand and offer congratulations. Often I have thought myself lucky that I am not royalty or a film star—how they cope with mobs of people continuously recognising them and staring at them, I do not know! I feel very sorry for them.

I remember once, when I was travelling on a bus, that the West Indian bus conductor recognised me and came up to wish me well. His natural flamboyance was so charming. He said: 'Man, I must put Gary Sobers first, but after him you're the greatest thing on two legs!' Well, of course, who could fail to respond to that? There was another occasion when a young man came up to me on a train and said that he and his mates had a bet on as to whether or not I was 'the heart transplant man'. I asked who had said I was, and he pointed them out, and when I asked who had decided I was not, he had to admit it was him. 'Sorry, mate,' I said, 'you've just lost yourself a fiver!'

Mind you, being recognised can have its disadvantages, too. When I

134

attend a charity function or fête, being on mild diuretic tablets and being unsure of the toilet facilities there, I usually find a public toilet and pop in there as a precaution. Two or three times I have been recognised in these establishments, and the ensuing conversations were usually of an identical nature.

Standing side by side in the stalls, faces are the last thing that people look at. When, eventually someone glances at my face, they automatically turn round and put their hand out for me to shake in congratulation. Instinctively I put my hand out in return and then realise that I was either trying to do my zip up to continue the ceremony of shaking hands, or that the two of us would be there, hands grasped in salute, baring all before us! Believe me, you feel a bit of a fool, especially when any other gentlemen in the toilet, on overhearing the conversation, come over to shake my hand with their own hands which had, not two minutes before, been used for other things! Clinically, it's a bit off-putting!

Now, to finish off the two months for me which could never be repeated, I'll describe the 1981 Papworth fête. The run up to this was that Paul Coffey had arranged a cycling tour from Wolverhampton to Papworth Hospital, with a few of the transplant patients arriving co-incidentally at the fête. We all agreed to take part. Gordon McDonald (another heart transplant patient) was going to fly down from Scotland and arrive at Gatwick. He would then travel by train to Victoria where I would meet him and we would both get the coach from Victoria coach station to Wolverhampton.

Now, Doreen and I are ordinary people and we soon discovered that we were well out of pocket, running all over the country to these various charity functions, and by that time our finances were in very bad shape. Reluctantly, we decided that we just couldn't afford to go to the Papworth fête that year so, when I met Gordon at Victoria, I took him to the coach station and told him there was no way I could come with him and that I would 'phone Paul with an explanation. Gordon didn't quite know what it was all about, but he went on his way with the message for Paul.

A few hours later, following Gordon's arrival, Paul was on the telephone: 'Keith,' he asked in a worried tone, 'whatever is the matter?' (He thought that I was ill.) I soon explained to him that it was just finance which was preventing Doreen and I from attending that year and I apologised profusely. He replied that he would see us at the fête anyhow, but again I explained that it was a 50/50 chance that we wouldn't make it, but I wished him and all the others all the best of luck.

Now, I presume Paul had got on to Papworth about this because, in a very short time, June, who was Secretary of the Papworth Staff Club, telephoned too. (She is also Secretary of our Transplants Club.) She explained that she was just planning who was going to do what at the fête and wanted to know what time I would be arriving. I told her that it would be a big disappointment to Doreen and me, but we just couldn't make it this year. There was a moment's silence and I sensed a bit of stand-offishness in her voice. 'Oh well, if you've got another thing lined up . . .' her voice trailed off. 'Oh no, June,' I said quickly, 'You know full well that I wouldn't attend anything else on a Papworth fête day. There's no point in beating about the bush—we're skint.' June said she completely understood.

Within half an hour, Joy, who was Chairman of the Papworth Staff Club, was on the 'phone. She asked what it was all about and I replied: 'Well, Joy, that's the way the cookie crumbles—I just cannot do it, and I don't want to get deeper in debt as it would take me ages to get out of the mire.' Joy asked if I could physically get up to Papworth. I knew what she had in mind and, because I dearly wanted to be there I told her that all I would accept was my petrol money to and from the fête. 'Just you get up here,' was her final order.

There is no point in having stupid pride, especially when one of your first loves is concerned, so Doreen and I decided to go. We duly arrived on the morning of the fête and went in to see June and when Joy appeared she had an envelope in her hand which she stuck in my pocket. I told her I hoped it was just my petrol money. 'No, it bloody well isn't just petrol money!' she exclaimed. 'In that envelope there's £50 from the Staff Club and, what's more, June and I are going to follow you two about all day and we will make sure that you spend every penny of it thoroughly enjoying yourselves. If you can charge round the country doing your bit for Papworth—then we can do our bit for you! We are,' she added, 'one big family here, never forget it!'

Well, that's one thing I have never doubted—I know Papworth. So when people ask me to do things for Papworth and Mr English or some other doctor gets a bit worried about me overdoing it—my feelings are how could I refrain from doing something for a hospital I love? This gesture from the Papworth staff left me overwhelmed. This was *not* a Ministry of Health hand-out, it came from the staff—the workers at Papworth who had done this for us. Well, I suppose you're thinking this sounds like a Hollywood tear-jerker, and to be honest I suppose it did make me have a few sniffles when the girls did it. So, we did enjoy ourselves that day. Harry Lowe came to the fête and even Percy, who I was surprised to see walking about already after his operation.

Eventually, the cyclists arrived, and a couple of nephews of mine, with two friends, who had done a sponsored walk from Bracknell to Papworth, came into the arena. That evening, the dance turned out to be a real cracker. This was a real red letter day for Doreen and me. I was sorry I missed the cycle ride part of it, because their first overnight stop on the journey was at *The Red Lion* pub at Brafield, which was the pub I visited after my release from Papworth and I had also judged a kids' Guy Fawkes parade there. In fact my Jackie travelled over to Brafield (her house is nearby) fully expecting me to be with the cyclists, and she was a bit surprised not to see me there. Well, once again all's well that ends well and, thanks to the girls at Papworth, Doreen and I were able to go to the fête.

10

A change of Panorama

By now, my poor old car was taking a hammering. It had developed oil pressure trouble when I visited my cousin Tony in Bracknell. For some reason, on my car the oil pressure seemed to affect the brakes and suspension as well. The following week I had similar problems with it when I was returning home from Bristol. I realised that I would have to start overhauling it. Unfortunately the spares were a bit expensive for this model but my cousin rang me from Bracknell saying he thought he had a bit of luck for me. He said that he could get his hands on a car which would only cost me £25! It was the same make, year and model as my present car—the going rate for it would have been £250 or £300— and would therefore have all the spares I needed and, he indicated, it might even be better than my own car! I jumped at the chance.

So Tony borrowed a trailer and towed the car to my house. We compared my present car, which was white, with the 'new' car which was red and decided that the white car had a better engine but the red car had far better features—it had a sunshine roof and tow bar—although the body was a bit rusty. I decided that I would rather work on the rust on the red car than strip and transfer spares from it to the white one. I worked on the cars for a few weeks and ended up with a white car, with red doors and a red boot which I had no intention of keeping, and a red car with white doors and a white boot which I was going to keep.

When we were invited to functions, the organisers never knew quite what to expect. Some expected an invalid to arrive in a wheelchair and others, who thought I must be very weak, arranged VIP car parking facilities so I wouldn't have far to walk. Doreen was becoming more and more embarrassed on these occasions by our old banger as we often parked beside some really beautiful cars, as you can imagine. There we were in our rotton old red and white thing—we used to slink out of it, hoping we wouldn't be seen!

I soon became thoroughly ashamed of the car, too, so, one morning, I got a tin of red lead paint and quickly sloshed it over the offending white areas. It didn't look too good close up but, from a distance, passed as a completely red car. Over the next few months we kept swopping bits from the old car to the newer one until, eventually, there was only the engine to be replaced which meant that I could ditch the old car and give the other one a good strip down and a decent coat of paint. I was quite optimistic at that time that I would be able to keep this car on the road for some time, even using it so much to attend functions, because I had plenty of spare tyres, etc.

One day, I attended a get-together of retired ex-matrons, sisters and senior nursing officers, with the current patients, at St George's Hospital. It was a really lovely afternoon but I had to dash off to get home by about 5.30 as I had to be in Norwich at about 8.30 that night because, the following day, I was to address the Norfolk Section at a Life Insurance Association meeting. I arrived home in quite a rush, wanting to bath, change, eat and then belt off to Norwich. While I was rushing around Doreen, a little bit apprehensively, said: 'Keith, I've got something to tell you. I don't know if you've noticed, but your old car has gone!' 'What do you mean—gone?' I asked.

Doreen explained that two chaps from the council had informed her that the car (the one I was stripping down) shouldn't be on the road. If it was there the following day they would tow it away and fine us. She explained to them that I was still using it for spares and I definitely wanted the engine. The men told Doreen they would take the car away and remove the engine for us, but they wanted about £30 for their labour. Doreen didn't know what to do and she panicked. The men kept emphasising the penalties of keeping a car on the road untaxed and, in the end, she let it go. However, our daughter, Wendy, took the number of their lorry. I told Doreen that she had fallen for the oldest trick in the book and, without doubt, these men were cowboys. Still, there was no time to discuss it then, as I had to get up to Norfolk. Everything would have to wait until I got back.

On the journey up, the red car began to make more and more noise. It seemed to be the bearings. Just a few miles short of Norwich, it broke down completely. This happened virtually outside the local police station, so I went in to explain the situation to them. They were very good and helped me push the car into a cul de sac where I could leave it safely until I had sorted things out. They said they would keep an eye on it. I then rang the Life Insurance Association to explain what had happened and they wanted to send a cab out to pick me up. I said it wasn't worth it and that I would thumb a lift. They were quite worried about this because, as I said earlier, people half expect me to be an invalid. They persuaded me to get a cab locally, which I did.

The gathering that evening was more or less a social one—the main seminar wasn't going to start until the following day. The local police had already given me the address of the nearest breaker, because I knew that's where the car was going to end up. I was a bit mad because it was only the engine which was giving trouble and, had the old car still been at home in London, it would have been worthwhile towing the red car back and putting the engine from the white car in it. Unfortunately, because of those cowboys, this was out of the question.

During the course of the seminar the next morning, one of the members of the Life Insurance Association came up to me and asked about the car. I told her it was kaput. 'How on earth will you manage in the future without a car?' she asked. I told her there was no question of me getting another car and that I would just have to confine my charity work to the London area. I had to admit it was a blow to me. She then asked me if I would accept a car from the Association if they had a whip round—they felt I was doing a worthwhile job which shouldn't have to end through lack of a car.

I thanked her from the bottom of my heart, but refused the offer. I explained that Doreen and I had made it a rule *never* to accept any money or gifts. I had just been a very, very lucky patient and we didn't ever want to be in a position where people would say we were cashing in on this. The lady said she half expected a reply like that and asked me if I would accept a car *on loan*. I thought about it for a while and decided that this was a very different thing from actually being *given* a car. At least it would mean that they would be helping me to carry on with my charity work, so I thanked her very much and agreed to the offer on those terms, if it was possible for her to arrange.

I got a lift back to London with one of the members of the Association that evening and the next day I telephoned the local council to see if they had indeed authorised the removal of my old car from the street and, as I suspected, they confirmed that a team of cowboy operators was working in the area. I reported this to the police and gave them the number of the lorry which the men had used. However, nothing happened, so I had to telephone the breaker in Norwich, giving him permission to break up my car. I confirmed this in writing and asked him to send me his bill. He very kindly said that, under the circumstances, he wouldn't charge me for the job. He also offered to hang on to any personal possessions he found in the car until I could arrange to collect them. Luckily, Roger, a friend from *The Fox and Hounds*, had to go to this area for a golfing week-end and he agreed to pop over and pick up my bits and pieces. How kind people are.

Doreen and I did try to get on with our charity work without transport, but it was very difficult. Public transport was all right if there was a direct route but, if the route was more tortuous, it took us ages to plan the journey. This was annoying as well as being too time consuming so we had to slow up on our activities.

Then came a really marvellous offer. The secretary of the Life Insurance Association telephoned to say that they had sent a circular letter about my car to their members and one of them had a car in the fleet which they would lend me. He gave me the name and address of this insurance company and asked me to telephone them.

I give this company full marks—not only were they offering me a car, they weren't doing it for the publicity. Their director told me that they had a 3-year-old Polo on their books and that they were only too pleased to lend it to me. They also gave me a £25 per month petrol allowance to keep me going. All *I* had to do was go and collect the car. Now I am going to give them the publicity they deserve—three cheers for *The Manulife Insurance Company of Stevenage!*

I travelled to Stevenage with the Secretary of the LIA so that Manulife could present the car to me—they even laid on a buffet lunch! I knew the car was 3 years old and I didn't expect it to be in a particularly good condition (the Fleet Manager had already told me that they would see to any maintenance or breakdown bills). However, when I saw the car, my eyes nearly popped out of my head—they had given it the valet service! It was absolutely gleaming and I was over the moon about it! I just couldn't find the words to express my feelings—everyone was *so* kind to me. It was seventh heaven driving home. Doreen was speechless, too, when she saw it, and we would like to take the opportunity now of thanking Manulife for this marvellous gesture. So, in a very short space of time, we had seen two different sides of people's nature as far as cars were concerned. Fortunately, our story ended happily.

Before we knew it, another Christmas (1981) was upon us, and the end of the second complete year of my new life was coming into view. We sat down and reviewed the past year. The first thing we noticed was the quickened pace of our lives—we spent so much time dashing about the country making public appearances that we didn't have much time for ourselves. It was a pity because it meant that I was unable to get back to the art group and my friends there. They understood. I didn't mind being thrust into the limelight but it was all getting too much for Doreen. She still had the house to run, of course, and Kevin was still at home, and we all know how untidy a schoolboy is! We also had to keep leaving Kevin, which certainly wasn't fair on him. Fortunately our daughter, Wendy, lives opposite us, and Kevin always knew that, if he came in from school and we weren't there (if we were delayed at a function), he could always go over to Wendy's, but it wasn't the same as having his parents about. Consequently, Doreen began to spend more and more time at home and less time attending functions with me.

Although the year was very happy for me, there were unpleasant moments, too. In the early half of the year both Harefield and Papworth really got into their stride with transplants and things were going quite nicely for them. However, the inevitable arguments over the ethics of this type of operation soon flared up. This is exactly what the hospitals didn't want. They just wanted to be able to get on with their job, but always there was something that threw them back into the headlines. It was all very unfortunate. People were now beginning to play the numbers game—'only so many have survived out of so many operated on'. This was entirely the wrong attitude to take, but this seemed to be the basis of their arguments. Looking at it from the other side, I soon found that there were more people who had died whilst waiting for a heart transplant operation than those who died after receiving one. The whole situation wasn't helped by a television programme, which I thought was rather irresponsible—*Panorama*. They did a somewhat sensational programme about donors in America. In it they claimed that many prospective donors were still alive when it came to the point of having their organs removed. Of course, this programme caused an absolute uproar in Britain, especially after the euphoria over the success of the heart transplants. The whole donorship programme was affected, particularly kidney donorship which was hit badly.

Spokesmen for the British Medical Association were offered the opportunity to reply to this programme and eventually they did but, to me, they were too gentlemanly in their approach, although through their knowledge of medicine and their logic, they managed to refute every argument on that programme. Unfortunately, the donorship programme has never fully recovered from this.

I met some patients from Harefield shortly afterwards and I explained to them that even in Papworth there was a certain opposition to the transplant programme and certain cardiologists were not supporting the surgeons as far as transplantations went. My friends couldn't understand it at all and were horrified to think that there were divisions of thought about it. Jim Kelly said: 'Well, Keith, at Harefield we find everyone pulling together.' I replied that in general terms so they were at Papworth. A cardiologist there did not believe in transplants and said: 'Let's not ape the Americans.' Fair comment, everyone is entitled to their views. Presumably, not apeing the Americans implied not duplicating effort. How glad I am that TE didn't sit on his arse and wait for further American results or I wouldn't be here now.

Now I didn't really want to discuss this in this book, but I do believe you get nowhere in life if you duck issues. What really upset me was that people criticized Papworth, the place I absolutely idolised. This is probably the only thing that has upset me since my operation. This was the year in which the number of transplants were increasing and many people were able to go back to work and justify getting a new life and the first mother-to-be had been given a new heart. Who could possibly knock this? Now, more than ever, I thought of the advice which Bill Ginks had given me—the best way for me to endorse the heart transplant programme was to get back to a normal life and be seen enjoying it.

However, as much as I tried to help, it slowly dawned on me that all the goodwill in the world could not buy the necessary expensive equipment for heart transplant operations. My main aim in life is to raise money towards this end.

Physically, the only problems I had this year were the ulcerations I got whenever I cut or grazed myself. (This is a side effect of the steroids I'm on.) My heart performed marvellously. In both cases, this is still true today.

11

Things get worse—but not the patients

By now, a year of intense sporting activity was beginning to tell on my bad right knee. Way back in 1951 I had had the cartilage out in the Rowley Bristol Hospital and, since then, I had suffered from arthritis. This was now getting worse and worse. This had nothing to do with my heart—although, of course, the new heart had allowed me to carry on with a bit of sporting life and so, indirectly, could have been responsible. There was concern about operating on this knee when I had to be immuno-suppressed. Anyhow, I feel that, if all I have to moan about during the last two years is an arthritic knee, that's not bad going, is it?

Naturally by now, Percy had been back home for a long time, and, on this particular Christmas (1981), something happened which just summed everything up for me. During the week leading up to Christmas, the local Rotary Club (Coulsdon) were collecting money, underneath a Christmas tree in the high street, for the British Heart Foundation, and I spent the week there with them. It was rather cold then so I was well wrapped up. I was just standing there, rattling my tin when, suddenly, there was a yell from the other side of the road and there was Percy Ayres—driving a lorry with a load of logs on it! We were *both* doing what we enjoyed most. I was raising money and he was back at work. The most important thing was that we were both leading normal lives. This was true of all my friends who had had transplants at Papworth. In that particular week before Christmas Paul Coffey was working at his hospital, Nigel Olney was busy getting on with his chiropody practice, Gordon McDonald was running his restaurant by a golf course, Andrew Barlow was again engaged in his engraving work—and I believe that year that Pam Dewar had gone to France for a holiday with her husband and child. It seemed to me that generally people were unaware that we had all returned to normal lives, and I did feel that it would have been nice if all those people who had been playing the 'numbers game' had known this.

Doreen and I had a lovely Christmas with several social events to attend. I wouldn't say it was quiet, but it wasn't hectic either, so we enjoyed ourselves. We had already been to record a programme for Pebble Mill for Hogmanay, and this was in the can. In fact we actually

144

spent New Year's eve at the Penta Hotel with the British Heart Foundation. Strictly speaking we were in two places at once!

The first few months of 1982 passed in the same way as the previous two years had, and we did a fair bit of running around. My only medical routine was attending a clinic at St George's every 13th week and once at Papworth every 13th week and these were so arranged that I was seen by a medical team every 6 weeks. In theory this was what should have happened but this sequence often got broken. Anyway, for social reasons, I was always popping in and out of Papworth.

Obviously, as a result of Papworth Hospital, East Anglia is a very special part of the country for me and we have been to lots of activities there. We often call into the hospital after some function to use the canteen there (this is the only café open on the road!) We always go up to the top floor and have a quick word with anybody who is in the Unit. On my clinic days I often bump into former patients and friends who are also attending clinics—we always end up swapping our symptoms like old ladies!

When I was first released from Papworth, I used to have ECG and blood tests at clinics twice a week there. I was then, obviously, a direct out-patient of Papworth Hospital but, by 1982, the British Heart Foundation had set up a Research Unit in the grounds of Papworth. This was a nice little Unit, consisting of several Portakabins, with Mr Cory-Pearce in charge. This is where I now go. So I wasn't really sure if I was an out-patient of Papworth or belonged to the British Heart Foundation Unit. I don't suppose it matters, obviously I was right on hand for the hospital should I need to be admitted for any reason.

As soon as the spring arrived it was time for Jock's fête, in aid of Papworth, up in King's Lynn. This year, Jock had really gone to town and organised a piano smashing competition! Four teams had entered with six men in each. Three of the teams were made up of healthy young men. The fourth team was from Papworth but, because of other engagements, only four of us could compete. When you consider that the combined age of the four of us was about 170 years and the other teams had *six* men in them I don't think we did too badly. I think the winning team smashed a piano in 4 minutes and some seconds and our team did it in about 6 minutes and some seconds! We certainly hadn't had any practice in breaking up pianos! For a bit of a joke we told the local radio commentator that Les, the convenor at Papworth, had been training us all for a world record and that he had been looking after us from the beginning to the end. When we told him that Les was the mortuary attendant at the hospital and was going to get us in the end, he looked absolutely aghast! It always amazes us that people find it hard to laugh at those sorts of things. We want to, and indeed have to laugh about death, what else could we do?

The most amazing thing about the fête was that I was to open it by being lowered down on a rope from a helicopter. I don't think Papworth was too keen on the idea, and the Ministry of Defence *certainly* wasn't, so instead it was decided that I would *land* by helicopter and not be lowered by one! A substitute helicopter had to be arranged as the original one was called for duty in the Falkland Islands and, with the wife of the Commanding Officer of the local helicopter station, I duly arrived to open the fête.

It was a bit windy that day and the pilot was a bit worried as to whether or not we could land. He warned that we might have to return to the station. When he saw the landing spot he was even more worried because, although the organisers had cleared a circle in the crowd, it wasn't a particularly big circle for a helicopter of that size to land and around the perimeter of the circle there were several tents, including my own old one. This old tent was a bit battered as, during my illness. when I had not been able to use it, we had lent it to several people and we had not really looked after it as well as we could have done, but we had put it up in order to use it as a stall at the fête and I was a bit apprehensive about how it would stand up to the down draughts of the helicopter.

As we came in to land, there was just a fractional tilt of the wings which meant that the down draught hit the ground at a slight angle, instead of being vertical. From the helicopter we could see a couple of tents lift up into the air, and to my own great amusement my tent stood the test well, despite its state, and the police tent and one of the fairground barker's tents both went up in the air about 20 feet! Unfortunately, one little girl was hit by a piece of hardboard which went bowling along the ground—I think it was just a shock for her and she wasn't hurt as I heard no more about her afterwards. I hope she was all right. Anyhow, the fête was a great success.

At this time, I found out that the main thing that Papworth needed was a gamma camera. This is one of those nuclear scanner-type things, with a computer read-out. It would be invaluable to the hospital's work. They didn't want, nor could they afford, a big one—a portable one would be more than ample for their needs. As far as I am concerned, if TE wants a gamma camera, then TE will have one. However, this would have to be a long term project because however enthusiastic you are about collecting, it takes a long time to raise as large an amount of money as that. I also realised that in 1982 there were a lot of charity events going on and the raising of the Mary Rose would naturally take pride of place over many other charities, so I decided that I could do little until 1983. But a rather nice thing happened then.

I had received a letter from an American student in London, Miss Tracey McLeod. She was doing a school project on heart transplantation and she wrote to me for some information. I telephoned her home to see if I could help and discovered, as I suspected from her letter, that young Tracey was only 10 years old. She asked if I could visit her school on Project Day, so that she would have a live exhibit!

Of course I gave her all the help I could and was delighted to visit her school. Without asking her parents or her teachers, Tracey and a few of her friends then went on a sponsored walk and raised just over £40 towards the gamma camera fund. So you see, young Tracey had really started the ball rolling and I got going earlier than I had intended. I think it is so marvellous that those young kids have worked so hard! So, throughout the rest of 1982, I continued to get the fund off the ground, though I planned that the main push would take place in 1983.

Papworth and Harefield continued successfully with their work during 1982 and many new people joined our 'Transplants' Club. One day, something happened which caused me a little embarrassment. It was hilariously funny though! I was taking a team from London up to a village near Papworth (Conington) to take part in a sort of mediaeval game called dwyal-flunking! This is now a pub game; it's great fun, and lots of beer can be downed should the competitors so desire! We were playing a team who billed themselves 'undisputed world champions'. It was all very tongue in cheek. On this occasion they were wearing sweat-shirts with their team name emblazoned across them. Not to be outdone, we decided to pop into Papworth and pick up our own sweatshirts, so we would look a good match for them.

Well, of course quite a few of the chaps who travelled up with me hadn't actually seen Papworth Hospital and were quite awe-struck when I took them all up to the top floor to get our shirts and get changed before driving the 3 odd miles to the village. I jauntily marched down the corridor with the others tiptoeing reverently behind me. Suddenly, I noticed the staff scrubbing down one of the Barrier Rooms and I knew what this meant. They were preparing for a transplant that day. The nurse confirmed this so, of course, I got the team out of there as quickly as I could, I knew they had enough on their minds without having to worry about what we were doing!

We arrived at our charity event and I saw Dee and some of the nurses on the Papworth staff. We had a great game—it was completely new to us—and the local Press took pictures of our antics. During the course of the game, Julian, a friend of my son, Kevin, told me that he had left his coat in the linen room at Papworth. (This room is where they store the sweatshirts and souvenirs which they sell at their fêtes.) I 'phoned the hospital and asked if someone could get the coat out of the linen room and take it up to the top floor where I would collect it on the way back to London. This they did, but now comes the embarrassing part.

The only sober people on the way home were Eddie, the driver, and myself—everyone else was well and truly carried away by the sporting activities and the resulting bevvying. As most of my lot were Chelsea supporters, they voiced their support for the club loudly, all the way to Papworth. 'Blue is the colour—Chelsea is our name . . .' they sang.

Once Eddie arrived in the car park I told him to try to keep everybody quiet whilst I went in for the coat. Now, on the top floor they had already started the transplant operation and there was I, trying to creep down the corridor and get out as quickly as I could, with the noisy strains of the Chelsea supporters drifting all over the grounds! In actual fact, at that very moment, Gillian Harris was receiving her new heart. I saw her a long time afterwards and she fell about laughing when she learned that she had received her new heart to the sounds of a football 'national anthem' and I am so glad to say that today Gillian is doing far better than Chelsea is!

In these days of sexual equality I still get a bigger kick from knowing that a woman has had a successful heart transplant rather than a man. I don't know why this is, I suppose it is because they are the ones who are then able to give birth to children. It always amazes me that many people seem to think that the operation doesn't work on women. I tell them that Papworth has done many successful transplants on women.

To me there was a slight disappointment at the Papworth fête of 1982. I looked forward to seeing more new faces as more people joined the Transplants Club, but I didn't get much chance to talk to people as I spent most of the time on our stall. I wanted to talk to some of them because once again the age-old argument between doctors at Papworth about the transplant programme had reared its ugly head. There was a lot of talk from the media about the Department of Health not financing Papworth and Harefield because they were now reaching a pitch where they were running out of money. However, I think a lot of people were just putting the Health Minister on the spot and trying to force his hand. Maybe I took a rosier view than some people, but I couldn't really see them withholding future funds. Obviously it wouldn't be a large amount of money as the country was in a bit of a mess, but I did anticipate some funding to enable the programme to carry on and I couldn't see how it could be stopped now as the success rate was too good. I had spoken to some of the Harefield patients about this, too, and I was asked by both Papworth and Harefield patients to be their spokesman about what we would do about the funding being withheld. Already some newspaper reporters had tried to put me on the spot with their questions, but I didn't want to get involved at this time as I thought it was the wrong time to rock the boat or predict any ministerial decision. On the other hand, we didn't want to be caught out on the hop and, as ex-patients, we all had our own ideas about what to do should the funding end.

I had taken some advice on how to react at this time and so I patiently explained to the other transplantees that we would not come out of it well if we made a great ballyhoo, but we would try to keep the programme going, although the charitable raising of money would be too intermittent to enable the programme to keep going on a normal course. We decided to hold our tongues and, later on, the decision was made to continue funding the two hospitals. At Papworth, we were going to run out of funds approximately three months or so before Harefield, so Papworth was given a slightly bigger grant to redress the balance. The two hospitals now will be running along on an even keel and they will both need further funding at the same time in the future.

Our minds were put at rest by this news, as we couldn't bear to think of the transplant programme being shut down. Luckily, we didn't have to put contingency plans into operation—we would have had to make a real ballyhoo to keep the hospitals open. We now hope that not only will there be adequate funding for transplants but that possibly, a new Unit will be opened in the future, perhaps in Scotland or somewhere like that.

All this talk of funding and the disagreements between doctors came at a time when I was first considering the fund-raising for the gamma camera, so it was very thought-provoking for me. As I said earlier, all Papworth basically wanted to do was to get on with the job in hand and not have these continual worries brought to the fore—moral and clinical arguments and now money—and I'm sure Harefield felt the same. Anyhow, they were now well geared up for transplants. Some people had left the team but others had taken their place and Mr Wallwork had joined Papworth to take over surgery from Mr English. Mr Cory-Pearce was in charge of the research side of things and Mr English was Director of the Transplant Unit at Papworth. Mr McGreggor was a very capable Senior Registrar (who has now left Papworth to do a stint in Stamford, California, which is the mecca for heart transplant operations). Mr Milstein is a very famous Senior Cardio-Thoracic Surgeon. Although he doesn't have much to do with heart transplants as such, he has given Mr English much support with all his work. Mr Milstein and I have had many conversations over the years and these days he usually greets me by saying that I am looking more and more like a bloated pig—as the result of my steroids affecting the size of my girth—but Ben always has a twinkle in his eye when he says it. The names I have mentioned above are only the top flight of the Thoracic Surgeons there, there are all the registrars as well and a marvellous nursing staff. I hope that the members of this wonderful team continue to see the fruits of their work.

The next major event, as far as I was concerned, was the Transplant Games to be held at Cardiff. By now my right knee was giving me a lot of trouble and I had difficulty in walking and, let's be honest, I was a bit too old to be a competitor. I did attend to help out with the Papworth stall. Not being a competitor, I didn't qualify for any concessionary fares or hotel rates and, in any case, I already had a commitment in London to attend a local school to judge children's pets. So, it was the Saturday afternoon when I did the pets thing in London, dropped Doreen back at home during the evening, grabbed my sleeping bag and put it in the boot of my car and drove off to Cardiff. I was going to try to bunk down in a friend's room in the hotel as again I was a bit broke. This duly happened and there was great hilarity when I smuggled the sleeping bag into the room, and slept on the floor that night!

Every time I saw the Harefield lot the same old question of the divisions between the doctors again raised its head. They were quite surprised when we told them that, as far as Papworth was concerned, the cardiologists had nothing to do with us now and it was all down to the surgeons and they were amazed as this just didn't happen at Harefield.

Anyway, Gordon McDonald won the gold medal for golf which was fantastic! It wasn't the first time that heart transplant patients had taken part in the games, two or three from Papworth had entered the year before, but it was the first time that the two hospitals (Papworth and Harefield) had sent a team. We were now united as heart transplant patients. However, again and again the conversation turned to the doctors' dispute. I told the lads that it was really sad to see poor TE taking such a lot of stick and it was beginning to show in his face. Quite justifiably we Papworth patients think the man walks on water, and naturally the Harefield patients have the same opinion about Mr Yacoub, so they were sorry when we told them that our TE was beginning to show signs of strain. What made matters worse was, just after the games when we returned home, one of the doctors at Papworth really hit the headlines by naming patients.

The first thing I knew about it was when, after midnight, one of the newspapers telephoned me and got me out of bed to ask what I thought about being named. I didn't know what it was all about and mumbled, some sleepy answer but half an hour later, there was another 'phone call from another paper with the same question. By then, I was wide awake, and I asked them for further details. They explained that patients were now being named in the arguments and I hit back rather angrily that we should not be involved at all. But this time, there was a subtle difference in the wording and it embraced *all* heart transplant patients, not just those at Papworth. Well, of course, the following morning I had a lot of Harefield patients on the 'phone to me, hopping mad and furious that someone was bandying their names about. They were quite prepared to start banging the big drum. Jim Kelly had already dashed off several letters to various newspapers demanding that they put the matter to rest. I persuaded him and the others not to get involved in the argument as I felt it would do us no good and possibly harm the programme, but the thing was now boiling up to being more than an academic argument, and the poison had crept in. For the next couple of days I went out on the golf course so people couldn't get hold of me. I couldn't walk much then, but at least I was out of the way because the last thing I wanted to do was to make comments and statements at that particular stage.

Soon enough an old familiar voice came over the 'phone to me. It was, of course, Percy. 'Who is this bleedin' fool who's calling us all steroid slobs—I'll go and punch the bugger on the nose to show him who's fit or not!' Well that was typical Percy! I burst out laughing, but I had no doubt that he would carry out his threat, as Perce had little respect for anyone who upset his applecart!

I giggled to myself over the following weeks, because soon it was time for Percy's next clinic, and he was building himself up to prove his physical prowess, but of course there would have been an enormous rumpus if he had succeeded. I still popped into Papworth often after having been to functions in the area and I spent some amusing hours geeing up some of the young doctors about Percy's forthcoming visit! They used to laugh, but somewhat nervously, and the only one who was very calm about it was Mr Cory-Pearce—he knew that he could handle Percy, although it would be a struggle. That, in fact, is what happened. It took him about two hours to calm Percy down and, as yet, Percy's threat has not been carried out! Mind you, I still got a fit of the giggles when I found out how many surgeons were missing on the day of Percy's visit—the load of chickens! Of course, no one wants to get into that sort of argument, but it is perfectly understandable that Percy, and others like him, can get the hump over it. Besides this, the Harefield patients were justified in being angry when they were roped into an argument concerning a totally different hospital. I also noticed that, when I was attending functions or giving after dinner speeches, this question often cropped up and I think it should never have got out of hand the way it did and any arguments between doctors at Papworth should have been kept within those doors.

My third MOT at Papworth (August 1982) came and went. The only thing wrong was that I was beginning to get a swelling in my groin. During my MOT Mr Wells confirmed that it was a swelling of the glands. Over the next few months, it started to get worse and, at the time of writing, there are very deep lines cut in my flesh and a swelling. It's a sort of athlete's foot of the nether regions! Anyway St George's are giving me a very thorough going over at the moment as it is obviously a side effect of the steroids—but apparently it is a bit unusual and they haven't seen anything like it before. I'm being looked after so well that I'm not worried about it.

The main side effect of taking the steroids is that I have got a bit of a 'pot belly'. I must admit that I am getting a bit sick of the good-natured gibes I get about having a 'beer gut' and having to explain the real reason for it. It would be nice to get rid of it as I have always been a bit self-conscious about it. I am on a moderately low dose of steroids (15 milligrammes a day) and I understand from my friends who are on this drug because of their kidneys that I wouldn't show any extra weight if I was on 10 miligrammes a day, so my next little battle will be to ask Mr Cory-Pearce if he would reduce my dosage. I don't suppose this is possible but I'd love to lose this little bit of extra blubber! I have already given up any hope of having my knee operated on. It appears that this is right out of the question—I certainly couldn't have a steel pin or any other foreign body inserted into it, so I shall just have to live with it. I'm not a defeatist, but a realist, so I guarantee that I shall be walking about next year even if I have a little fat gut!

By now my fourth new Christmas was upon us—1982. We had a very nice quiet time at home doing absolutely nothing but putting our feet up. Mind you, I was a bit sore underneath, but that didn't stop me enjoying my Christmas. New Year came and, like the previous year, we spent this at the Penta Hotel with the British Heart Foundation. On doing our usual yearly review, Doreen and I decided that nothing untoward had happened—it was more or less the same as the previous three years—still rushing about doing our charitable work and having the usual medical checkups and, apart from this skin trouble and my knee, there was nothing wrong with me, but I was still unable to get to do a bit of painting with the art group. The only cloud on the horizon had been the doctors' arguments gradually brewing up.

We are now into 1983 and the main thing that I am involved in is raising money for the gamma camera. Many people are helping, too. This year Jock had his annual fête on the bank holiday at the end of May and he managed to get permission for it to take place in the Royal grounds of Sandringham. Naturally, as it was held on the Crown Estate, this fête generated a lot more interest. Jock had organised a mini marathon and The Caravan Club brought their members en masse. Jock has been spending the last few years learning how to handle these events and we are really thrilled that everything went well for him.

Dear old Jock, he cannot do things by halves and this time he asked if I would open the fête by flying in standing on the wing of an aeroplane! Even *I* knew that this would be impossible—not that I would have minded trying it—but I knew TE would definitely put the stops on that one. The Eddie Kidd jump a couple of years ago was risky enough as far as TE was concerned!

The very latest nice thing that has happened to me so far in 1983 is that the Manulife Insurance Company have lent me another car—it's two years old with only 12,000 miles on the clock. They have also increased my petrol allowance to £30 per month. People mistakenly believe that life assurance companies are in the business of trading with death. How many firms would make an offer like that—*and* shun any publicity? I can hear you critics talking about tax allowances, etc, but Manulife don't *have* to do it. I'd like to bang a little drum for this company and, as far as I am concerned, 1983 will be 'Manulife Year', because without them I certainly couldn't get about the country the way I do to raise money for Papworth and other charities.

Well, now I am up to date with my story. As I write this, I am approaching my fourth MOT! What hopes and fears have I? Fears? None! Hopes? Plenty! The only unfortunate thing that has come out of all this is the fact that it has been wearing Doreen down. I think now that she has felt more pressure in the last three years than she ever did whilst I was waiting for my operation. Gradually I am trying to shelter her more and more from all these pressures. I wonder if she feels that if something went wrong now there would be more to lose. To me there now seems to be so much bright hope for the future—after all, whilst we were fighting in those early days, there was no talk of heart transplants and so death was inevitable.

You know, in talking about death, I can now understand more fully why six million Jews could more or less passively face death in the gas chambers. It's not a question of being conditioned to death and its inevitability, but you do become rather tranquil about it if you allow yourself to. I can't really describe or understand this passive acceptance of death, but it can easily come to you. However, I have always been a fighter and will not give up my life without a fight. Looking back over my experiences, I think the worst enemies you can have when you are really ill are a passive acceptance or an over-active imagination. Passive acceptance means that you are just going to sit back, do nothing and let death take over, and an over-active imagination can be devastating. You must be optimistic and start to fight back—you will find that you have won three-quarters of the battle.

As far as my hopes for the future go—I naturally want the heart transplant programme to continue. Most certainly, before this book is published, a combined heart *and* lung transplant operation will have been performed. As far as I know, they are all geared up for this. I think Mr Wallwork has already performed this operation in America and, to me, it is the next logical step. However, I sincerely hope that, when the first person undergoes this operation, he or she will have less publicity over it than I had. I hope this patient is able to return to a normal life— that is what the whole thing is about.

Unfortunately, normal life is out of the question for me now. Although I really enjoy my charity work, and will continue to do as much as I can for Papworth, my private life has most certainly suffered and, in particular, I do regret the pressures on my wife. So, I wish the best of luck to the first recipient of the heart and lung transplant operation and I hope he will be able to settle down and enjoy his new life with as little fuss as possible.

Perhaps Mr English could have a calmer time too. At the moment he has been rejuvenating all of us at the expense of ageing himself with all the intermittent battling. I hope that in future he can have more time to himself. However, at the time of writing these words, the wretched doctors' arguments have started all over again and these are far more vitriolic than ever before. It will be impossible now for us patients to keep out of it—after all, I don't do things by half measures. From now on, we will start having our say over whether or not it is right that transplants should be done and whether or not patients should influence medical decisions. We have been drawn into the arguments now and we will be heard—we live in a free society. Of course, if we do kick back, our opinions will be biased, after all we know the full merits or de-merits of the whole question. We see friends of ours who become critically ill, have transplant operations and then lead new lives. We know how we feel ourselves. Surely if we don't know the success story then nobody does. That *Panorama* programme was bad enough, in my opinion, but I only hope that this argument going on now won't crucify the continuance of the heart transplant programme. Look at it from our point of view. We are, after all, human beings as well as heart transplantees and it does hurt to hear all this controversy about us. Some people have even accused us of being pawns in a medical experimentation game. If we are, then we certainly captured the queen first time. It is very difficult for us to sit passively, biting our tongues, with all these arguments about cost and morals going on around us.

I remember, back in 1979 when I first went to Papworth Hospital, that on the top floor the metal windows were so corroded with rust that they wouldn't shut properly. The builders came in and chipped away the high points of the rust and got back to the bare metal so that the windows would close but, to this day, Papworth Hospital haven't had the money to have them painted. They are now getting more and more rusty. It's the usual story of spoiling the ship for a ha'porth of tar.

12

People

I would like to end my story talking about the various people who haven't been mentioned so far in the book. After all, the British medical profession relies so much, from top to bottom, on unified medical teams and each person is as important as the next. It has been impossible to bring each and every one into this story.

One important person who is very much part of my story through his connection with Harefield Hospital and who I have only mentioned once, briefly, is Eric Morcambe. Eric, of course, is famous and best loved for being our favourite comedian. I first saw Eric on Jackie's farm, not long after I was released from Papworth. One of the London evening papers at the time was producing a colour supplement and they thought that it would be nice to show the two of us larking about as, of course, Eric has had heart trouble too. When his car came up the drive, we were all in the sitting room in front of a blazing log fire. The door opened, we all looked up expecting to see Eric, but no, a hand slowly came round the door waving a pair of horn-rimmed spectacles! It was Eric's usual funny entrance and we had a good few laughs although our grand-daughter, Sammy, let us down right from the start when she said to Eric: 'Oi, don't you lean on the mantlepiece, my mum's only painted it this morning 'cos you were coming!' The other funny thing happened later on. The paper wanted to take some photos of Eric and me sitting on the white fence which surrounds Jackie's paddock. Well, Jackie, being a natural bodger, had painted the fence with emulsion paint instead of the proper stuff and, as it was a damp day, the paint became a bit tacky. We didn't dare tell Eric that, through sitting on the fence, a bit of white paint had got on the back of his trousers and he was walking about like that! We hoped he would find out when he got home and wouldn't realise where it came from!

Later on, at various functions, I saw Eric, still doing his clowning. During one visit to St George's, I went up to Drummond Ward to see some of the patients there. One of them was waiting to go down for heart surgery and was thrilled to bits because he had received a note from Eric. He showed it to me—it wasn't one of those typed letters with a brief signature, Eric had actually taken the time to sit and write personally to this chap in his own handwriting and I thought it was marvellous that a busy man like him had taken the time and trouble to do this for an unknown patient.

I haven't mentioned Dr McGarvin. He worked in St James's Hospital and slogged his guts out to save my life on the night when I first arrested. I don't know where he is now, but wherever he is I wish him well because he is a fine doctor and I have a lot to thank him for.

Now, working with Dr McGarvin at that time was Dr Bellamy, who I have talked about. I didn't tell this story though. During a recent clinic I had to have a barium meal. I noticed that the pretty young lady doctor who was conducting this test was called Dr Bellamy. I said to her: 'Dr Bellamy, have you any other relatives in the medical world?' She grinned and said: 'Yes I have.' I then asked if this relative had any connection with St James's Hospital. 'Yes,' she answered 'my husband treated you many years ago and, funnily enough when I told him last night about my seeing you today, he wondered if you would remember him.' 'Who could forget him?' I replied and that little incident made my day because that was the second husband and wife team that I had met.

In the other couple's case, I met the wife first and then the husband. In the early days (when I had been considered a terminal case at St James's) it was time for me to come out of hospital, I put my head around Sister's office door to say: 'Ta ta'. In the office was Dr Wendy Rynance on her own. She said goodbye and wished me luck. It must have been very difficult for such a pretty young girl to have to try and conceal from me what she knew about my chances of survival—she knew I was being sent home to die—but she managed it. Months later I was treated by another Dr Rynance and I asked him if he was married and soon found out that Wendy was his wife!

There must have been hundreds of nurses, sisters and medical staff who, over the years, have looked after me and I would have liked to mention (and thank) them all, but this is impossible, however they can best be represented by Charles Hubbard, the Senior Nursing Administrator at Papworth. He is so delighted about the success of the heart transplant operations and he is also pleased for all of us. Many times Charles has volunteered to attend charity events if one of us transplantees couldn't, and he was always willing to help us in our fund-raising activities. He is a marvellous man.

I must also mention Les Simmons, the Papworth convenor, at this point as he also does a lot to help us raise funds. Les is always the first to volunteer to help. I remember trying to repay his kindnesses once when I was attending Papworth for one of my MOTs and there was a strike on. Les and some others were on picket duty on the gate, with nothing to eat or drink so, for a bit of a joke, I got some left over bacon from one of the food trolleys, stuck it between two pieces of stale bread and took it down to Les! The lads asked if I had come to join the picket, but I replied: 'No, but I felt so sorry for you I've brought you something to eat,' then I brought out this tattered old sandwich. Les's language was unbelievable! However, there was a good rapport between us. I wasn't taking any sides in this strike—these people were all good friends of mine. Anyhow, for me, Charles and Les seem to represent all the hundreds of staff I came across during my illness and recovery. I wish I was able to thank them all, although I know they don't seek recognition. As I remember Bill Ginks saying to me years ago when I tried to thank him: 'It's all part of the job to us.'

Then there was Woggie. Woggie was so ill himself and I didn't even know it for months and months. He was so good at giving me little bits of information to encourage me. I know his wife and children couldn't speak English and his wife was concerned that, if anything happened to him, she and the children would have problems, so he took them back to the Middle East. I do hope I bump into Woggie again, even if it's only to discuss with him a little story that Andrew Thorpe told me.

Apparently, one day Andrew picked up one of the magazines which were lying about the hospital rooms—it was *Penthouse*. While he was looking through it, he saw Brit, the new Senior Nurse who had just joined Papworth, walk in. Not wishing to be caught with a *Penthouse* magazine in his hands, he quickly put it into Woggie's lap saying: 'There you are, Woggie, you're looking for houses, see if you can find any penthouses in there!' Poor Woggie was left holding it when Brit introduced herself to him. But that's why I love them all so much—my doctors can tell me *their* jokes as well. They are all genuinely good people doing a wonderful job, and they enjoy a good laugh, too.

Somehow, although Andrew has left to do a 3-year stint in the Midlands, I still have the feeling that one day we might see him back at Papworth—and that goes for David Cooper too. Talking of David Cooper, I once asked Andrew this riddle: 'Why is TE like a busted barrel?' Answer: 'Because he is knackered without a good Cooper!' I don't know whether Andrew ever passed that on to either TE or Mr Cooper, but I am sure if he did they would have had a good laugh.

Another name which springs to mind is that of Pam Rhodes, the London Weekend Television newscaster. Pam is virtually the Papworth mascot from the days when she used to be with Anglia Television and used to do a lot for Papworth. She too, is very willing to help us with the fund-raising for the gamma camera.

There are so many people throughout the world who do all the nitty gritty work when it comes to charities. Their only reward is their sense of achievement; they don't want to be officially recognised. We all know people like that.

There are also the donors' next of kin—they have made donorship possible. What can I say about them? They are the givers and we are the receivers. They are the people who I feel most for when controversial TV programmes like *Panorama* cause so much hurt. After all their sadness and unselfishness! My feelings towards them must be obvious. Many of the donors' relatives still support us all they can. Many of them turn out for events to help us keep the donor programme going and, I am glad to say, that our relationship with them is very strong indeed.

And of course there is TE himself. What can I say about this man? Well, I will not say much about him personally, he wouldn't like that, (everyone knows I think he walks on water) but he is the most important doctor who has ever looked after me. I know I'm always blowing raspberries at him and the other doctors, but this is purely from the joy of living. I revere every single one of them, even those who criticise the transplant programme—criticism is good and I know well that, if I was in difficulties, these doctors would work their guts out to save my life, as they would for any other patient.

So that leaves only one person for me to talk about. I have tried not to say too much about her. Of course, it's my Doreen. I unashamedly say, and I have always said, that I have been blessed with a perfect marriage. It has been a good one. Throughout all our ups and downs I don't think we have had more than 25 rows in any one day! Sure, before my illness and when I was fit and well, she would give me a good telling off if I went over the top in some way, but that was quite natural. I would go as far as to say that Doreen's actions during my illness couldn't have bonded us together any more—it was perfect bonding in the first place. But her courage was wonderful. When I was very ill, lying on the couch all the time, vomiting into a bowl, day after day, she still had to look after the family—it must have been hell for her. There was all the embarrassment when we went shopping and I had this distressing vomiting to cope with and there were all the times when she was so worried about me that she had to tiptoe up to me to see whether or not I was still breathing. She must have wondered what the future held for her. I never ever heard her complain. I have only ever seen her cry twice—once in the Intensive Care Unit at St James's and the other time on the steps of Papworth when, with all the emotions of joy over my discharge from the hospital, she cried in front of the Press—but surely she can be forgiven for those two occasions.

Now, that it is all over, I still see her struggling to cope with this goldfish bowl existence which we have and I can see that gradually her nerves are going and she is smoking more and more—it's got to the pitch now where I have had to start bullying her to cut down. I am not going to ask her to give it up, I smoke myself but I only do it when I fancy a cigarette and don't smoke from habit. Throughout all our problems, Doreen has been fantastic. She has never complained, questioned or pressurised me. She left all the decisions to me but we have always pulled together in our marriage. She is always close by, not pushing me, but being totally supportive. Her attitude has rubbed off on all our kids, especially on Kevin, the youngest. At least all the others were old enough to understand that I had had a good run at life and, if it came to the crunch, well, that was that. Now Kevin was only 9 when all this started, and by the time he was 12, he had a lot to face up to—successfully, I am glad to say.

So, let me close this book with a few words about another love in my life—Fulham Football Club! I must confess that it was watching them that gave me a bad heart in the first place! I would like to think that when I go eventually (and that will be in many, many years' time) that bits of me don't end up in little bottles in Papworth's laboratory for, like all true football fans, I would like my ashes to be spread over the grounds of Craven Cottage. I would like them to be spread on the pitch before a really good match. Unfortunately, knowing Fulham as I do, within two seconds of the match starting, those silly sods would only slip on the ashes and concede an own goal—and then I'd never rest in peace.

The Keith Castle Gamma Camera Appeal

Keith Castle, Britain's longest surviving heart transplant patient, is raising money for a Gamma Camera (scanner) for Papworth Hospital. This scanner will increase the effectiveness of the diagnostic work at Papworth.

Please contribute generously, send donations to:

**Papworth Hospital
Papworth Everard
NR. Cambridge
Cambridgeshire**

Cheques payable to:
Papworth Hospital Medical Equipment Fund

This book is due for return on or before the last date shown below.

Don Gresswell Ltd., London, N.21 Cat No. 1208